LIVING
FULL

LIVING
FULL

Winning My Battles with Eating Disorders

Danielle Sherman-Lazar

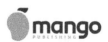

Mango Publishing

CORAL GABLES

For permission requests, please contact the publisher at:

Mango Publishing Group
2850 Douglas Road, 2nd Floor
Coral Gables, FL 33134 USA
info@mango.bz

For special orders, quantity sales, course adoptions and corporate sales, please email the publisher at sales@mango.bz. For trade and wholesale sales, please contact Ingram Publisher Services at customer.service@ingramcontent.com or +1.800.509.4887.

Living FULL: Winning My Battles with Eating Disorders

Library of Congress Cataloging
ISBN: (p) 978-1-63353-874-0 (e) 978-1-63353-875-7

Library of Congress Control Number: 2018957577

BISAC category code: SEL014000, SELF-HELP / Eating Disorders & Body Image

Printed in the United States of America

To my beautiful daughters, Vivienne and Diana. May you always be happy, healthy, and FULL *by every definition of the word.*

Also to the millions of people affected by eating disorders. You are not alone, and recovery is more than possible—stay strong. You are entirely capable of living a FULL *life.*

Table of Contents

Foreword

Eating disorders are frequently misunderstood. Adolescents and young adults affected by disorders such as anorexia nervosa or bulimia nervosa may struggle with self-critical thoughts and engage in potentially dangerous behaviors, without recognizing that they are living with classic symptoms of a serious psychiatric illness.

Danielle Sherman-Lazar's *Living FULL* is an honest description of one woman's battle with an eating disorder. Danielle describes the anxieties and obsessions that may have made her vulnerable to developing the pattern of food restriction and disordered eating behaviors that characterized her eating disorder, and the turning points that allowed her to achieve her recovery.

Her words are moving and authentic and reflect the loneliness of living under the cloud of illness and the liberation that comes with recognizing that eating disorders are treatable and that life without illness is possible.

As Danielle explains, eating disorders are brain-based disorders that are associated with serious medical and psychological disturbances. She sheds light on the importance of effective treatments, and the support systems, including family, that may be needed to achieve successful outcomes.

As a psychiatrist who has specialized for nearly thirty years in care for individuals with eating disorders and the study of the mechanisms underlying these conditions, I feel privileged to have played a small part in this tale of one person's recovery. I am aware of how difficult it is to reveal the many thoughts, doubts, and secrets that contribute to the development of an eating disorder. Readers will likely find parts of themselves in Danielle's tale, and find themselves inspired by her story of strength and resilience.

Evelyn Attia, MD
December 2017

PART ONE

Empty

CHAPTER 1

The Little Engine That Couldn't

I woke up to a crowd of kids and counselors surrounding me, my thick, curly hair forming a pillow behind my heavy head. My eyes blinked a few times before opening completely, vision hazy. I felt a breeze on my exposed skin, a warm one, but it didn't stop the goose bumps from forming on my arms. My gaze made its way down to the green pavement beneath me. Then the realization: I was flat on my back on the camp basketball court. *Oh no, please don't be real life!* Then the voice: *It is real life, and I am taking over yours.*

After a short trip to the infirmary, it was decided that I needed to go to the hospital to get an IV. I was mortified that my parents would have to take a three-hour car ride to make sure I was okay. I wanted to tell them they didn't have to—that I was fine—but I had no say in the matter. What if they figured out what caused me to end up in this state? What if they uncovered my secret? *Our secret.*

As far back as I can remember, I was nervous about mostly everything. In fact, there's hardly an anxiety-free memory I can recall. I was afraid Chinese ghosts possessed the ancient armoire standing prominently in my bedroom. It was decorated with Asian figures in different poses, embroidered in gold, from the Han Dynasty—that's at least what I concluded after watching *Mulan*. I was convinced their ghosts were angry Huns, not at all sweet and friendly like Casper the Ghost. I was also always scared that someone would break into the house. Every little squeak and creak made me leap and check under the bed for burglars or *worse*. In kindergarten, I became petrified of the tooth fairy and swore to my parents that I saw her in my room leading a marching band of fairies the night I lost my first tooth. They told me not to tell the other kids in class that I'd seen this so-called tooth fairy rendition of *Alla Marcia* because that might be seen as, in my mother's words, "a little strange." Oh, and perhaps I was too young to recover the next day and have the knowledge and wherewithal to blame it on a fake bad acid trip. *Yes, definitely too young.* So I didn't, out of fear that all of my peers would laugh at me—another *fear*.

Because of my anxiety, I was very attached to my mom. I hid behind her legs so often she joked that I would climb back into the womb if I could. I think she was right. But what she didn't know was that out of all of my childhood fears, it was the fear of people not liking me that kept me awake at night.

By the time I got to third grade, I had managed to make a best friend, Elizabeth, and fell in love with the idea of going to sleepaway camp with her. I played a lot of soccer, and hearing about camps that promised full days focused on sports was an unbelievable dream for a tomboy like me. Sitting beside a giddy Elizabeth, as the yellow school bus pulled away from my parents for the first time in my life, I should have felt excited. Instead I began sobbing, palming the filthy windows, mouthing to my mother, "I changed my mind!"

"Dani, run, we're in the lead!" shouted one of my teammates in the relay race.

I ran as fast as I could across the field, buoyed by the bounce of the fluffy ponytail one of the counselors had made for me.

The baton no longer my responsibility, I took a seat on the sidelines, sipping water from the bottle labeled "Dani Sherman" in my mom's handwriting. I traced the words with my fingertips, trying to keep my concentration and catch my breath. The heat had hit me hard and I was sweating from parts of my body I didn't know had sweat glands. I heard cheering around me, but it was disorienting. I couldn't wait for this race to be over. All I wanted to do was sprawl on my bunk bed and close my eyes. I felt so weak, drained, and light-headed from sprinting—feelings I had never felt before. I usually loved the adrenaline and competitive nature of races. Today was different. This race drained me. I heard cheering around me again, but this time it was even louder than before. We had won. I feigned excitement to appease my friends, but I was really just cheering because I was closer to lying down and that made me *really* happy.

I started walking back to my bunk with one of my friends. Her curly hair was in a high pony as well, and she had a peppy bounce in her step, matching her Slinky-like bobbing curls.

"I think the gold team has a good chance to really get ahead of the green team at the swim meet, don't you think?" She was chatting about Color War, the highlight of the camp session.

I nodded.

"We have Michelle on our team too, and she is the fastest swimmer in our age group and..."

Suddenly, her mouth was moving but I couldn't seem to make out the words. It was like someone with a remote control had pushed the mute button on our conversation. Was that buzzing in my ears? My vision faded in and out, in and out. Then, everything stopped. Was I dead? I must have been—everything was black, and I couldn't move. Suddenly, I was in my bed at home sleeping soundly, warm and safe with my mom and dad right next door, the way I liked it. I could hear my mom's voice trying to wake me up and felt her hovering above me. Why wouldn't she just let me sleep? "One more hour, please, Mom." I sleepily begged, "I am so tired. Fine, ten more minutes. I'll compromise..."

"Dani, are you okay?" *A husky voice was far away but getting closer—maybe Mom had a cold?* "She's okay, step away, and give her air." *Wait a minute, that wasn't Mom.* I opened my eyes and, to my horror, I was right. It wasn't my mom; it was the basketball instructor, and there was a crowd of kids, counselors, and instructors—way too many people for my liking—surrounding me. I had fainted.

The camp owners, the counselors, and the campers murmured to one another their theories on what had caused me to faint. I was like the top story on E! News, Summer Sports Camp Edition. I was the talk of the camp, the big gossip of the day. Even after I returned from the hospital, pumped with saline and sufficiently hydrated, everyone wondered, was it heatstroke? Is she sick? Only I knew the truth: I'm starving.

It began on the first day of camp. I was beyond consoling and wanted only to be back home. How would I find comfort without my mommy and daddy? At dinner, I scanned the food stations, piled high with mac and cheese, meatloaf, hamburgers, hot dogs, and baked beans. It just all turned me off, which was odd, because I had never felt that way about food before.

All of the choices overwhelmed me. I put some mac and cheese on my plate, but no, I didn't really want that. I then rotated my head, making sure no one was near, and scooped it into the garbage, then put a hot dog bun on my empty plate. I didn't want that either, back to the garbage. Repeat. Besides completely wasting food, it was agonizing and embarrassing all at the same time. I wanted to call 911: "Police, please, I can't seem to make a decision and I am about to have a panic attack. I can't choose what to eat. Yes, you heard me right. What to put into my mouth." Instead, I just stood there, doing this little dance between the buffet of food and garbage until I wound up with a simple peanut butter and jelly sandwich (this was before peanut allergies were a prevalent thing, and something called "peanut butter" was offered with jelly at summer camps and school cafeterias nationwide). Panicked in the face of so many food choices, and afraid someone would notice and make a citizen's arrest on behalf of wasted-food-kind, I became known as a picky eater. Every day that summer, I consumed:

Breakfast—Raisin Bran with skim milk

Lunch—One peanut butter and jelly sandwich

Snack—Nothing

Dinner—One peanut butter and jelly sandwich or a cheese sandwich

Snack before sleep—Nothing

There was no deviation. The camp had a kitchen staffer make me a sandwich for each meal. When my bunk was called to get food, I would go off on my own through the double doors leading to the kitchen. Peter, who ran the kitchen, would bring me my sandwich, and I'd take it back to the table where my bunkmates gorged themselves on French fries and tapioca pudding and sloppy joes. With each bite of soft white bread, I'd savor and swoosh the sandwich in my mouth. I knew I couldn't eat again until the next meal, so I had to hold on to each mouthful as long as I could. Everything was new—living on my own, meeting new people—but the sameness of my food numbed me like a sedative, dulling the homesickness, the social anxiety, making me feel more at ease.

When I began to lose weight, it was noted that my activity level surpassed my nutritional intake. To try to counteract what was happening, the infirmary made me have Carnation Instant Breakfast once a day to help keep my weight stable, but that didn't work. While campers were getting their morning medicines, I was getting a waxy paper packet of vanilla calorie supplement. I allowed myself to break my newfound diet regimen because the flavor reminded me of home, of Saturday afternoon milkshakes with my mom and dad at TGI Fridays after a soccer game. Done with the performance anxiety—the pressure I put on myself to play well, to be the best on the field—I treated myself. To make it last longer, I poured only a tiny splash of skim milk in, to make it into a pudding-like substance instead of a drink. I would then scoop each bite into my mouth as slowly as possible, savoring it so long the packet would sometimes last for an hour.

I was like the little engine that couldn't. The day I fainted, my train had to use its emergency brakes. I didn't have the fuel to go on anymore the way I was, and my body broke down. Revving *choo choo* no more, my small train officially derailed. The counselors, and even the doctor at home, had seen this happen before. A very active child in summer camp tended to lose weight. The truth was, I was always hungry, but I needed my patterns and rituals much more than

I believed I needed food. Plus, I was over my big caboose holding me back.

FULL LIFE, MAY 2013

Sitting in front of a blank computer screen, I tapped my pencil twice on my desk and slipped it behind my ear, pulling my long thick curls behind with it. I wanted to make a difference so badly but was not sure how.

WHERE IS MY PLACE? I wrote in big bold letters on the paper in front of me and then placed the pencil back behind my ear.

There must have been a reason I survived. I needed to tell the reason I am here and not in the ground, dead—to help other people struggling. Too morbid for a Facebook post?

I had decided to raise awareness by doing the first thing that came to mind that has reach—make a Facebook page. I wanted to mobilize people toward a shared goal of physical and mental FULLness; I called it Living a FULL Life, but so far I had posted nothing. Except for a profile picture: me, hair in a tight bun, smiling wide, pointing to the lettering on my blue shirt—"Nobody's Perfect" in thick white letters. I wanted the page to raise awareness about eating disorders by inspiring others to live a FULL life—a life that is centered on physical, mental, and emotional health, with an eating disorder in the rearview mirror, because it is possible.

Well, here goes, first post ever...

I have known my intention with this page but have been trying to figure out how to go about it. I want to help fight the stigmas surrounding eating disorders: they are self-imposed superficial diets and are all about being as thin as possible. FALSE! I think it is important that people should NEVER live in shame about their struggles and know they can ask for help with no judgment. Eating disorders are a disease like cancer, I was once told by a professional on the subject. However, people remain "in the closet" on this topic because of the negative stigmas. I think the best method to recovery is to share your story, own it, and let others know that they are not alone and can live a FULL life without their ED. I think my personal struggle with anorexia and bulimia wouldn't have gone as far as it did if I had known this.

Also, we live in a skinny obsessed society. It's time to accept people of all shapes and sizes and know that you are beautiful for who you are. No one is perfect, but you are a perfect version of you. There is no one else in this world like you and that is amazing. Let's fight this battle together.

I clicked Post and sat back in my chair.

What is living a FULL life exactly? Having anorexia or bulimia, or vacillating between the two, you are emptying yourself or trying to achieve an empty feeling through starvation or purging. Living a FULL life is a life where you aren't starving anymore—starving for acceptance and love from others and yourself. It's a life where you are feeding your mind and soul with good thoughts and foods. It's a life without your eating disorder. With our eating disorders, we are empty of opportunity, growth, challenge, and possibility. Living a FULL life means filling up our lives again with immense potential, happiness, and achievement.

It's a life where you make mistakes, and you are not hard on yourself for those mistakes. A life where you are self-aware enough to go against your negative thoughts and outside your comfort zone and are able to make healthy decisions. It's a life where you are able to nourish your body and soul with nutritious and delicious foods, and fuck it, if you want dessert, you are going to have it and not think twice. A life where you can beat your eating disorder at its own game of shame, guilt, and manipulation and realize that life isn't a losing battle. Your battle is just a small part of you; it doesn't define you. Once you beat it and own it, so you are held accountable to yourself and others about that struggle, you will become immensely stronger and well on your way to being FULL.

This book is that journey.

CHAPTER 2

Hello, Anorexia

Just as the doctor had predicted, back home in the fall, everything went back to normal. I was eating without limitations and with variety again and got back to a normal weight: a weight approved by all adult parties. The weight gain didn't bother me all that much. I was at home, surrounded by sameness and by people I loved. The soothing effect of starving was no longer necessary.

But once I got to sixth grade, that need to control would come back with a vengeance, and my parents being around would not be enough to keep the ED voice at bay. *You can't silence me forever.* Actually, voice, yes I can, but I wasn't quite there yet…

With the change of schools from elementary to middle school, and the quadrupling of my class size, nothing was predictable anymore.

Elizabeth was already dieting, munching on baggies of celery and slices of fat-free Kraft Singles while the other kids gobbled up trays of greasy cafeteria pizza. This confused me, as I thought she was gorgeous already, with her long straight brown hair and feline cheekbones, but her mom was the kind of health nut who thought yogurt was a proper dessert, so I guess I shouldn't have been that surprised.

In many ways, Elizabeth and I were opposites. Elizabeth was naturally bright, even though she chose not to apply herself, while I had to study very hard in order to get the As I craved. That's because, when I was in third grade, I was diagnosed with a processing problem, meaning it took me a little longer to absorb information than most students. I remember that conversation very well.

"Your dad and I were talking, and we think…. Well, what I am trying to say is maybe you could use some extra help." My mom paused, fiddling with her fingers trying to find the right words. I saw they weren't coming easily to her—maybe she could have used some *extra help* for that. Come on, was this really so embarrassing to talk about that she couldn't even find the words? Apparently. "We decided to hire a tutor to help you with your reading comprehension."

"Why? Do you think I am stupid?"

Of course she thinks you're stupid.

"Of course not, Dani. We just don't like to see you struggling, and this could make school easier for you."

You are struggling because you are a complete idiot.

From that moment on, "You're a failure" became an internal mantra: Why couldn't I be as smart as everyone else? Why did I have to work twice as hard to do just as well?

My tutor was my secret, my processing issue was a taboo subject, and I made it my mission to study extra hard to camouflage what I believed to be my natural stupidity. I learned how to work around my processing problem in class by becoming a speedy and precise note-taker. Frankly, I was hardly listening, just writing everything down, knowing I'd go home and study it all slowly. My classmates noticed, and I'd get calls at home asking to copy my homework or to look at my notes. Sometimes twenty calls a night. My mom threatened to pick up and tell the kid off, but I'd secretly call back and give the answers. I knew I was being used, but I liked to be needed. I was pleased to be so good at something that people took notice. They needed me, and, if they were going to like me, hell, my inner people-pleaser would help them, their mother, and their dog too, if he would lick my face in the midst of tail wagging (you get it, I'd help anyone—animals and humans alike—if they would give me *some* positive reinforcement.)

So I continued to take studying and school very seriously, while Elizabeth was off having fun, because she could. While I was busy fielding questions about the social studies homework, Elizabeth was flitting about a new kind of social event: boy/girl parties. The kind of parties where kids *drank*. Once, I went with her, and watched with fascination as she placed the edge of a beer bottle cap on top of a table, holding the neck of the bottle tight, and used her other hand to slam down on the bottle as the cap went flying off. How did she even know how to do that? I still slept with stuffed animals and collected antique Snoopys as a hobby.

"Want a sip?" Elizabeth asked, after taking a long chug.

"No, thanks," I said, backing up so much I tripped over a multi-colored beanbag love chair behind me and fell next to a boy-and-girl duo flirting, teasing each other, and touching. The boy rubbed the girl's back, leaning against the beanbag—that now had me on it too. I tried to gather my wits while interrupting their intense chitchatting. They started giggling as I grazed one of their Solo cups, catching it before it fell, joining in on their laughter because, in that embarrassing moment, my nerves got the best of me. Heck, what else was I supposed to do?

I felt like Alice forgetting Tweedledee and Tweedledum were alive, because, gosh, those flirters looked like waxworks at that moment—they got so still after our awkward laughing session. *Kill me now* was the only thought I could muster.

"Suit yourself," Elizabeth whispered under her breath as she walked toward a group of older boys—eighth graders—leaving me to recover from my own clumsiness.

"Thanks for helping me up, Lizzie!" I muttered, apologizing to the flirters while pulling myself up and planning my exit from boy/girl party hell. But, despite her rudeness, I was in awe of her. I could never have that self-confidence and ease around people. That cool way of being that seemed to come so naturally to her. That was the first and last party I ever went to with her.

Despite our differences, I loved Elizabeth like a sister, and I envied her edginess and rebellious nature. I loved sports, while she liked theater and art. I called her my "artsy-fartsy" friend. She liked makeup and boys and, during our play dates, she would stare at herself in the mirror, applying different colored lipsticks while jabbering about which boys in our grade were hot. I did have crushes too, only I was too shy to speak to them unless I was playing sports, baseball cap backward on my head, ready to kick their asses! Elizabeth already had boyfriends. I actually spied on her first kiss; it was outside my house by a rock I would later dub *the kissing rock*, which was hidden at the edge of my family's property. It was famous as a make-out spot for Lizzie as she took all her boyfriends there throughout our years as friends. In addition to her straight dark brown hair and dark blue eyes (a killer combination), she was slim and tall. Plus, she developed early, and was already a C-cup by sixth grade. *That lucky bitch,* I thought.

Walking into school with Elizabeth, I felt like her furry little pet. "*Woof woof,*" I imagined students barking at me as I passed. "No treats, please, I'm watching my figure," I'd say back. And as if to seal my furry-pet status, kids called me Fluffy, on account of my kinky brown hair. It was humiliating. Every time I heard it, my eyes would tear up and I'd hold my breath until it passed. Who would want to date or be friends with Fluffy? Answer: no one. I would eventually spend an hour each night before bed with a straightening iron, slowly bringing each unruly strand under control because of this *awesome* nickname.

Every morning, Elizabeth would take absolutely forever getting ready for school. She would do her hair, apply makeup—all the girly activities I had no interest in. One morning, when Elizabeth's mom was late picking me up in the carpool to school, I was more impatient than usual. It was the last day of school, so I didn't have any last-minute notes to study and distract myself with because there were no exams and grades were already finalized. Actually, there was no point in going to school at all, except to keep up my perfect attendance record.

It was unusual for camp to start so quickly after school ended, but we were leaving for it the next day. I wasn't excited, I didn't want to leave my mom and dad and the comforts of home. Except I knew I needed to work on my soccer skills and other top-secret goals. Because lately there was something else bothering me. I'd started to take notice of my changing body for the first time. Suddenly I had curvy hips and a round bottom, thighs that jiggled when once they'd been taut as trees. Fat. Fat. Fat. Disgusting.

While I waited for Elizabeth's mom, I glared at myself in the mirror. Why did I have such a big butt? And my thighs, ugh! My stomach was getting so big! Scowling in disgust, I vowed that summer I would lose all of my puberty weight and become even skinnier. Then I would feel better.

"Dani, Lizzie and her mom are here, where are you?" My mom's shout echoed through the vents in the bathroom. Dani had been my nickname ever since I was a little girl. My parents and those closest to me knew me only as that...and Fluffy. Lucky me.

"Be right there, Mom!" I shouted, deep-breathing in. *One more day...*

"Have a great day, Dani." My mom kissed me on the cheek and handed me a brown lunch bag, which a quick glance revealed to contain a tuna fish sandwich, yogurt, and two chocolate chip cookies. Usually I'd just eat the yogurt and nibble on half a sandwich, but no longer. All I could think was more thigh fat, butt fat, stomach fat—*fat, fat, fat*. I kissed her back and stuffed it into my backpack. She would be so disappointed and confused if she knew I was going to toss it into the girls' room trash.

Dinner at my house was not a family affair, so I never had to worry about *not eating* there. It wasn't like in most of my friends' families, where I heard rumblings about *togetherness* and *grace before meals*. I imagined something out of a 1950s movie—the mother cooking and the father demanding his steak medium rare with a side of buttered mashed potatoes—and the child sitting with her legs crossed, napkin placed neatly in her lap, and talking about her day while politely declaring, "Oh, shucks" if she dropped her fork. No, that wasn't our house. All of us had hectic schedules, so family dinners were pretty rare. My mom stopped cooking once I got picky and "stopped appreciating her efforts" (direct quote). "I would never, not appreciate your scrumptious meals!" I'd retaliate, deadpanning. In my defense, Mom wasn't a cook.

So we ordered in every night from different places. I would usually pick at whatever I got in the computer room while doing homework. After soccer, this athlete had little time for chitchat while refueling—I had a processing problem, for God's sake! I needed to study! That excuse let me eat—or not eat—as peacefully and privately as I liked. My dad and mom would usually do something separately when he got home from work. As much as they didn't act like it, in other ways—in the romance department, for instance—they were the cute 1950s adorable lovey-dovey couple that actually enjoyed each other's private company. And it wasn't even vomit-inducing for my snarky preteen self; I loved witnessing their solid foundation.

But there was one thing my mom and I always did together—late-night snacking before bed. We usually chatted about our day as we nibbled, munched, and nibbled some more. So later that last day of school, my mom and I were munching on cereal straight from the box for dessert. This evening I had Cinnamon Toast Crunch and she had Honey Nut Os. I was starving, since I'd skipped breakfast, thrown out my brown-bag lunch, and only picked at dinner, trying to start my diet pre-camp. It's hard to sleep on an empty stomach, so I usually gave in to the hunger pangs during evening snacks. Plus, the comfort of hanging out with my mom, my best friend, sealed the deal.

"I am so full, I need to stop. I am getting so fat," I said, loosening the waistband on my sweatpants, trying to relieve the pressure of my expanding tummy.

"Dan, no you aren't. You always lose weight at camp anyway," my mom said, putting a Honey Nut O into her mouth.

"Well, I need to!" I exclaimed, popping a piece of Cinnamon Toast Crunch into my mouth. "You see, I can't help myself," I added. "Ugh."

My mom chucked a Honey Nut O at my head.

"What are you doing?" I laughed and threw a handful of Cinnamon Toast Crunch in her direction. It hit her right in the face, leaving a cinnamon and sugar mark on her cheek. "Bull's-eye!" I screamed, hands waving in the air declaring my victory. We laughed so hard that my stomach hurt, or it could have been from eating too much, but either way, I knew one thing in that moment—I was going to miss her. I was going to miss this.

"I am going to miss you so much," I said, making a pouty face while sitting back in my chair.

"I am going to miss you too, but camp will be so much fun." My mom had loved sleepaway camp in her youth. She went until she was the oldest age allowed and was even a counselor for some summers afterward. I wasn't sure camp was my thing like it was for her. Even though Mom was my best friend, we had very different personalities. Everything always seemed to come much easier to her than me in the friends and fun category of life. She had the face of a model and a flawless body. A personal trainer and spin instructor, my mom was a walking billboard for the classes she taught. She was perfect, and I was...well, I couldn't even compare. I just needed to go to camp to lose weight, to get everything back in order. I was out of control. Look at me over here, stuffing my face with Cinnamon Toast Crunch.

"Yeah..." I trailed off.

"I am going to miss walking in on the two of you this way," my dad interrupted our powwow, entering the kitchen from his office, taking a work break by pouring himself a big glass of milk.

That night, my dad's wild curly hair was tight against his head with a thick coat of gel—dark black with slight salt on the edges. He likes the gray because he thinks he looks distinguished, and he does. My dad is a tough businessman and an extremely hard worker, with a huge personality and a confidence that is both awe-inspiring and intimidating. Yet he is a family man and has a big, generous, sensitive heart that even manages to break at every Disney movie, including *Aladdin* and *The Lion King*. I mean, gut-wrenching sobs, inducing thick tears down his cheeks, which no one would suspect based on a first impression.

"I was just saying that. It was like you read my mind," I finally spoke, coming out of a trance—eyes focused straight ahead at nothing in particular.

"Mark, why don't you come sit with us for a bit?" My mom said, pulling out the seat next to her and patting it, gesturing him to come.

"Okay, Linda, but I only have five minutes. I have a big meeting in the morning I need to prepare for."

"We are going up to bed in less than that anyway."

As my dad sat down, finishing his glass of milk, and their chatting continued, I put my hands on my stomach, sizing it up. This was the last time I'd binge on cereal. Tomorrow at camp would be the start of my diet, no slips ever again. Tonight was the last night of late-night eating and talking with my mom. This *really* was the last time. I pinky-swore—and a pinky swear means business. I'd never break that pact. *Yeah right!*

And I was right about that, at least for that summer. I became more engulfed in my eating patterns and rituals than ever before. A lot of it had to do with my vow, but also with the fact that I hated my new camp. Elizabeth had switched camps to one that was coed and supposedly more down to earth, with kids from all over the country, not just the Tri-State Area. Of course, I'd followed her. Also, in the old camp, more and more girls in my age group were becoming more materialistic. It was a fancy camp, and what clothing brands you wore and how boys responded to them at socials mattered more than people's personalities. Material things never mattered to me. Look, I grew up in an environment where I became acutely aware of nice things and even brands (guess I am a byproduct of where I came from in some ways), but I never base anyone's value on having those items. I also never needed or wanted those things; they were just always around me, so I became attuned to them. So even though I befriended a nice group of girls, I still found myself feeling more and more homesick for Mom and Dad. I thought trying something new, maybe a new environment, would be the cure. I was wrong.

Unfortunately, the new camp wasn't any better for me. My homesickness was at a magnitude of 9.5 on the Richter scale (meaning *whoa high* like the Great Chilean earthquake of 1960) and dieting became my only reprieve. I'd stopped eating peanut butter and jelly sandwiches when I became aware that peanut butter was fattening. So it was jelly only, on whole-wheat bread. Maybe that was the giveaway. One of my counselors noticed my food peculiarities and reported me to the head of the camp. Thereafter, my counselor was instructed to watch over me to make sure I ate every fattening morsel on my plate. It was humiliating, because my bunkmates knew why I was being monitored. At the time, our bunk was split into two groups—the new campers and the old campers (think *West Side Story's* rivalry between the Jets and Sharks)—and the old campers would whisper and snicker to each other about my eating problem.

Each bite I took was a mouthful of shame and worthlessness. To help keep my weight up, my mom sent protein bars to the infirmary, where I was sent after each breakfast to be forced to eat one and then get weighed. Again, at dinner, I was forced to eat my entire meal, followed by a second trip to the infirmary for my second protein bar.

When visiting day arrived, I only had one thing on my mind: my escape.

"Please take me home, I hate it here," I begged, eyes swollen from crying.

What was the point of being at camp if: (a) The camp was all "hippy dippy" and "kumbaya" with no focus on sports, and (b) I couldn't lose weight anymore; in fact, with the amount they were *making* me eat, I was bound to gain weight. I repeat, *gain weight*. And, in my distorted mind, I didn't have a pound to spare. Yes, as Queen Bee (Beyoncé) would say, ring the alarms! I needed to get out of this hellhole like yesterday. I needed to go home.

"But Dan, you love camp. I think you just miss us, and we miss you too, but this is where you will have more fun," my mom said, as she wiped the tears off my face with a tissue she pulled out of her tote.

"No..." I tried to find the words to explain, voice breaking. It was *so* much more than just homesickness. They were making me shamefully eat in front of my peers, stand on a scale and *see* my weight rise, and pointing out my problem for all to gawk at. Until now, my eating patterns had been my private secret—or at least no one had confronted me about them, trying to *help me* by counteracting all of my hard work.

"Dan, you have your best friend here. At home, you will have nothing to do," my mom countered.

I stood there speechless, tears falling onto my hair and soaking the top of my T-shirt, nose leaking into my mouth.

Then Elizabeth—who, being my polar-opposite best friend, normally didn't get emotional—interrupted our conversation, taking my hand.

"Dani needs to go home," she said, her blue eyes filling with tears. "She's miserable here. Please take her home."

That must have been enough to show my parents that this was serious, that it was more than just homesickness.

With that, we packed up all my belongings and were off. Nothing more was said about it, at least until we got home. Then my mom was all over me, peering around every bend with her snooping eyes:

"Dani, is that all you are eating?" "Dani, what are you doing for dinner?" "Dani, is that enough?" "Dani, please let me make something for you." *Kill me.*

Oh, and if I wasn't embarrassed enough about having a tutor for my processing issue, it was because I was never told I'd have to start seeing a therapist. Never, that is, until now. That's the confirmation I needed to prove that I was a total wack job. Mom, not being familiar enough with eating disorders to realize what was going on, was worried about my anxiety issues and why I was so unhappy at camp.

"Dan, I found a therapist for you and I am taking you to your first appointment tomorrow."

"Okay." I was so happy they'd let me come home, and I didn't want to ruffle feathers. If it made her feel a little more at ease and kept her off my back, I was completely *okay* with *said shrink* for *said wacko.*

While previously my weight had gone up during the school year, then down at camp, then up again by fall's end, this time I kept to my diet, and I was heading into seventh grade skinnier than when I had been rescued from camp in July. What differed is that this time I went into the camp experience with a poor body image triggered by my perfectionism, rather than homesickness. Homesickness can be left behind at camp. These new problems? Not so much.

In late August, when Elizabeth got home, my mom and I met with her and her mom for lunch. I ordered my staple favorite to appease my mom: chicken fingers with French fries. When the order came, everyone dove into their food while I carefully picked at the chicken fingers, trying to get beneath the fried batter to the white meat, while I quarantined my fries to the edge of my plate.

"Dani, stop this, and eat your fries. You like them!" my mother ordered.

You know when someone holds their breath to the point where they feel a head rush, and then they finally exhale—panting and breathing maniacally? Well, she basically couldn't hold her tongue anymore, which led to an *explosion* of words: "What are you doing to yourself? You don't need to lose another pound. What do you want to do, disappear?"

Actually, I never considered that, but maybe—disappearing sounded so magical, like poof and abracadabra, then you are gone... no more worries. How blissful.

Elizabeth and her mom looked at me like I had five heads, six limbs, and acne on every inch of my skin. But that didn't worry me as much as the fact that I had made my mom mad. I grabbed the dinkiest fry from the banished pile and ate it. That was honestly the best I could do.

"Look, I am eating, are you happy?" I whispered, trying to shift the attention elsewhere by being discreet and quiet, making light of what she'd just brought to the attention of the entire freaking table—thanks, Mom! Mindset: if I brush it off, they will too. Yes, discretion. Clearly my mom wasn't familiar with that concept.

Elizabeth's mom was an extremely healthy eater, or at least a dieting pro. In fact, she was quite helpful simply by example. By observing what she ate, I had learned that French fries were in the "bad food" category, something I'd never considered before. I learned what "good" foods and "bad" foods were, according to Diet 101, Elizabeth's Mom Edition, at least. "Good" foods were any type of steamed and plain or "dry" fish and chicken, salad with no dressing, vegetables cooked without oil, and egg whites. The "bad" foods were basically too numerous to list, but the general rule was absolutely no carbs, which meant avoiding pizza, fried food, Mexican food, anything ethnic that wasn't steamed, and so on. Basically, anything that tasted good.

As an impressionable and insecure middle-schooler, all I knew was that Elizabeth's mom was beautiful, smart, happy, confident, and thin. She had it all together, the answer to everything, and on top of that, she fit in. Oh, to have her confidence and ease around people. I wanted a fraction of it. If I dieted, maybe I could have what she had.

By the time I turned thirteen, I became hyperaware of the bodies of girls and women around me, including my own mother. People told me how much I resembled her, which I thought was utterly ridiculous. "Yeah," I'd say with sarcasm, "I'm the troll version." My mom didn't like it when I said that, but I had proof! When the movie *American Pie* came out later that year, I became known as the Shermanator (a loser character who loved Terminator movies) to my peers, while my mom was voted, by the same peers (thank you, horny middle-school boys!), number-one MILF (Mom I'd Like to Fuck)—the only social honor I'd be remotely associated with, by the way. She thought that was gross. I thought it was *way* better than being the Shermanator.

I had a one-track mind and continued to be meticulous about what I put in my mouth, when, and how often. My weight was slowly decreasing, but not to the point where the doctor my mom took me to found it concerning.

"Linda, she is really active. I really don't think anything is wrong. This has been happening since she was little," the doctor said, adjusting his thin glasses onto his slightly crooked nose.

"I know, but I am just making sure, because she seems to be watching herself lately," my mom said in a low voice.

I wanted to scream and signal with my hands, "Yoo-hoo, Mom, I can hear you. I am right here," but I refrained.

"Dani, is this true?" I felt the doctor look at me, his big brown eyes like spotlights. He knew me so well, having been my pediatrician since I was a baby. It was hard for me to lie to him. Hard, but not impossible.

"No," I quietly answered, twisting my curly brown hair into a bun on top of my head and wondering how I could similarly twist this conversation.

"Then you won't mind if we add milkshakes to your diet to help you gain weight?" he inquired, as if testing me by my reaction to his request.

"As long as it's vanilla," I instinctively blurted. "Can I have that instead of vegetables?" I added, trying to sound like the naive child they hoped I was.

And BINGO, they *loved* that answer. My mom and the doctor were both satisfied with my fake childish request, but, the truth was, all I could think about was how I was going to compensate for those shakes.

They didn't know how good the empty pit in my stomach felt. They didn't know how satisfying it was to have control over one damn thing in my life. I couldn't control how hard it was for me to keep up academically without anxiously studying 24/7 or what people thought of me, and *gosh* it gets tiring trying to please *everyone*. In fact, nothing seemed to come naturally to me but *this*— dieting. And I wasn't going to be the one to let them in on my secret, that it was deliberate, especially when they were so intent on taking it away from me.

To placate my mother, I drank those awful milkshakes twice a day to gain back some of the weight. After just a few weeks and pounds gained, my mom let me go back to "regular eating." She even stopped watching over me, thinking I must be fine. The physician hadn't said I had an eating disorder. GPs weren't as aware of identifying and responding to eating disorders as they are now. Eating disorder awareness and knowledge of it as a mental illness wasn't as widespread back in the '90s. He just said I should gain a couple of pounds and, once I did, that was that.

Aside from observing how thin or heavy other girls my age were, I decided to try "fitting in," and started to pay attention to what popular girls did and wore. At thirteen, I began straightening my hair with a flat iron every night. I started to wear tight jeans and even tighter tops. Thanks to the skinless, juiceless, tasteless chicken I had eaten over the months, I finally felt confident enough in my body to wear something besides sweatpants. I began putting on eye makeup in the morning, carefully curling my lashes with a metal device that looked like a torture implement.

Surprisingly, I managed to fall in with a group of girls who were considered popular, Elizabeth included. Even more surprising, I got my first boyfriend. We never spoke. Actually, our breakup talk— initiated by me—was our longest conversation during our entire daylong relationship. The reason I bailed: his previous girlfriend implied I'd have to make out with him, and my inner perfectionist shouted, "What if you are a bad kisser?!" I couldn't risk it and was too terrified to go through with it. Overall, really skinny seemed to be treating me well, at least from an outside perspective.

As I fried away my frizz for hours a night, thinking, *Take that, Fluffy,* Dani Sherman was changing. Yes, I was changing my look, but my desire to fit in was tested by the biggest change of all.

Books like *Are You There God? It's Me, Margaret* make getting your first period sound exciting, something to be eagerly anticipated. But really, is there any rite of passage more humiliating? At least that's how I felt. Everything about this change into something unknown to me—*a woman*—freaked me out. First, the act itself was disgusting—like *ewww gross*, a horror movie in your panties. Second, this intensely mortifying gross experience is somehow *never* private. I decided I could avoid some of this by not telling my mom. So I concealed the blood, using tissues as pads. Reality check: tissues last only so long. I needed parental guidance to tell me what to do to stop *Scream 4: Panties Edition* from staining all of my clothes.

"Mom, I think I may have gotten my period," I blurted to her the next day, tears dripping down my face. I wanted to disappear.

"Oh wow, congratulations. My little girl is growing up. Wait, you think? Are you bleeding?"

"Yep!" I shouted between sobs.

"Why are you crying? This is great news."

"I don't know," was all I could say, through broken tears and heavy breaths.

My mom, having gotten the confirmation she was looking for, put her arms around me, holding me tightly. Ugh, teary-eyed and huggy. Like, please, anything but *that reaction*. And, as I predicted, everyone wound up finding out: aunts, uncles, cousins, my father. The very moment when I most wanted to crawl into bed, hide, and never be noticed by anyone in the outside world was the same moment that all attention was on me, with mazels and the Jewish *minhag* (ritual) of the slap in the face—and that slap hurt!

Then no sooner did my mother bring home my first box of pads than I got boobs. Does anything scream, "Look at me!" more than two protruding knobs of flab? I was becoming a woman, except I could never compare to the women around me, like my own mom and Elizabeth's. They belonged in this upper-class town, and there was one thing I knew for certain—I sure as hell didn't.

I was different from this town and privileged life I grew up in. I didn't belong here, and I hated it. I hated the fact that it was so hard for me to find my place, to fit in, to be normal. I hated the fact that I felt so different—so weird—and I couldn't put my finger on why. But most of all, I hated myself for hating it so much. I knew these were lucky problems, and how dare I feel bad about myself when there were so many *real* problems in the world? I also felt like I could never do enough to make up for all I was given. I would never be enough.

I calmed this guilt and self-hate with the only control I had, control over food. This meant further tightening the reins on my eating, thinking the less I ate, the better I would feel. I would chew on Cotton Candy Bubblicious instead of eating breakfast or lunch. Every single night, I would order steamed vegetable dumplings or steamed chicken or shrimp with mixed vegetables with no sauce. I would savor each bite I took. Even the blandest dish tasted like heaven to my starved palate.

I liked eating my one meal in private because I could take my time and really savor each bite. After I was done, I would still have a twinge of hunger in my tummy, and that would make me feel satisfied. I would play soccer every day after school, and while I was running, I wouldn't only think about being the best on the field, I would think about all the calories burned, and about how when I sweated, my stomach skin would get cold. Someone told me that meant you were burning calories, so I would always feel my stomach for that coldness and smile a little when I touched it.

I decided to stop pretending to be a cool, normal girl. *Normal?* I could laugh at the fact that people actually believed that farce. Normal people don't think about ways to lose weight 24/7. Normal people don't have to study into the early morning to keep up. Why should I even try to fit in? It was making me stand out and be noticed in ways that I didn't feel ready for—like my daylong bogus relationship and comments about my cool clothes, which made people take notice of what I believed to be a not-good-enough body. Plus, caring about my clothes and makeup wasn't me. I was over pretending. I didn't know what *me* was, but I was trying too hard to be something I wasn't, and it was getting tiring. I started wearing baggy sweatpants again (let's be real, comfort always mattered more than style to this girl) and tossed my makeup. Every day after school, while girls made plans to go to the mall or head to each other's houses to do their homework, I went straight home, put on my back brace for my bad posture, which I hadn't told a soul about, not even Elizabeth, and did my homework alone.

"Why don't you hang out with us anymore?" Elizabeth asked between classes in the hallway one afternoon.

"I don't know. Just been busy," I mused, then changed the subject. "So, my darlin', in more important news, what's going on with you and Robert?" I gave her a nudge with my elbow.

"Well, we were at this party, playing spin the bottle..."

Worked like a charm. Deflection, deflection, deflection.

Going home alone also allowed me to avoid the after-shopping group trip for Chinese food at Tea Garden, where I used to get sesame chicken. There was no way I could eat that anymore, with its sugary sauce and pools of oil. It was hard enough to make excuses about lunch. If I stayed with the group, how would I skip what had been my favorite dish? That deep-fried and battered chicken that had once made me salivate now made me want to gag.

The girls were changing anyway and not for the better. Boys, parties, and material things seemed to take priority over anything, friendship included. Those topics were bullshit to me, and I preferred to spend time alone then be bothered with it. Looking back, I would have felt this way anywhere I went to school. There are good people and bad people everywhere, especially at that impressionable age when people are discovering who they are—and simply put, baa—kids become sheep and are easily swayed in their opinions, sometimes doing the wrong things just to fit in. I wasn't comfortable with what they were about, but I also wasn't sure what I was about either. I couldn't handle the bad kids—the kids who were mean and made fun of other kids—and most of the good kids were like me: shy, unsure of themselves, quiet. I couldn't navigate and find my own friends while dismissing the mean girls around me.

That's why I decided I'd rather focus on things I could control: my diet, sports, and schoolwork. That's what truly made me happy, or at least protected me by keeping me safe from experiences and people that could potentially hurt me. For the rest of seventh and eighth grade, I lived like this—waking up from anxiety-ridden nightmares about heading to high school, where things were sure to get lonelier and much more complicated.

My fears were right. When high school began, I was left with soccer, homework, and my eating disorder—the only friend I could trust, the only friend I could count on, and the only thing I could control.

FULL LIFE, SEPTEMBER 2013

"Are you feeling better?" my dad asked as I entered our shared office. I saw the big fish hanging on his wall. My grandpa had caught it many years ago, and it had been hanging there ever since, back when he and my dad shared this same office. I stared at its majestic dark blue fins and light blue scales—*Such a nice contrast,* I thought.

I work with my father running a fleet of taxicabs. My great-grandfather started the business, my grandpa and dad each helped build and expand it, and I am the fourth generation and the first female to come in and help run the show. Following in my dad's footsteps was what I had wanted to do since I was twelve, even before I knew what his job entailed. All I knew for certain was that I wanted to "take care of my entire family," like I had seen my grandpa and father do.

"Better, thanks," was my reply after coming back from my little brain tangent. "I am just having a sad feeling day." I paused, trying to clarify what that means. "Just not feeling great." I took off my black winter jacket and hung it on the back of my chair. I sat down, making myself comfortable at my desk.

"I know. I'm glad you came in, though. I need a lot of help here," he said, scrolling through his emails. He knew I should get out of bed, and that's why he'd made such a stink about my not being in the office that morning. He did it because he was afraid to leave me alone and depressed again after everything that had happened.

"I feel better now after I forced myself up," I said, trying to make him feel better. Also, it was kind of true. I felt better after getting my shit together, forcing myself out of bed, brushing my teeth, attempting to brush through the thick knots of my kinky hair, getting fresh air. It all helped to some degree.

"Good," he replied, and turned back to his emails.

I decided to write a post to help other people who may have felt like I did:

> Some days when every flaw on your body and face becomes detectible. Some days when you feel insecure and anxious. Some days, you want to close your eyes, go back into bed, and pull the blanket over your head. Some days when you are forced to do something out of your comfort zone which is everything, besides the warmth of your blanket, seeming so convenient and safe at the moment. Some days when you have these destructive feelings about yourself invading your body—penetrating your soul. Try to remember you are a visual representation of how you feel on the inside, not what you see on the outside. Get out of bed, smile. Laugh at your original self-doubt and conquer the world. You will feel better and maybe even beautiful despite yourself.

Now it was time to get to work. I had a ton to do

"Here it goes. Today, I conquer my work; tomorrow, I conquer the world," I said under my breath, knowing that everything was going to be okay. I had taken the hardest step. I got out of bed.

CHAPTER 3

Hello, Bulimia

My premonitions about high school were spot-on. Elizabeth kept on having fun, flirting, and making new friends, while I spent the first two years wrapped in my schoolwork, soccer, and, most of all, dieting. Strangely, I never knew how much I weighed. I feared the scale because I knew it could trigger a downward spiral. Not being under one hundred pounds would be a disaster, so why torture myself? I was a pragmatic anorexic.

Once in a while, I would slip and eat more than I should, and when I say more than I should, I mean I would stuff anything in sight down my throat. Then, feeling horrified, self-hating, and completely out of control, I would try to throw it all up, but I couldn't. I would gag over the toilet until my throat hurt and my eyes were teary. Slamming the toilet seat in frustration, I would hate myself even more. What kind of idiot can't even puke? One-word answer: *me*. To compensate, I would work out extra-long the next day.

I was pretty good about sticking to my diet, but because of those occasional binges, I didn't lose an excessive amount of weight in a short amount of time, which helped me stay under the anorexia radar.

By the summer before my junior year, self-control was no longer winning out. So I found what I thought was the answer to my dieting prayers: Laxative bulimia.

I know, *cringe*.

We were in Nantucket over the summer and I had been constipated for a couple of days. Anyone who has ever experienced constipation can vouch—that shit (pun intended!) *hurts*.

There I was, fifteen years old and running down the soccer field. I had terrible cramps and could hardly breathe, but that wasn't stopping me. *No!* I was so determined to play well for my team, I kept going in what felt like slow motion. Suddenly, though, I became so overwhelmed with chest and belly pains I couldn't go on. *I'm having a heart attack!* Subbing myself out, I sipped water while sprawled on the green grass, awaiting death. To express the pain properly, I can now only use acronyms because there was too much discomfort to form actual words: OMG (oh my God) and FML (fuck my life), to put it mildly.

My parents, seeing my distress, quickly bundled me into the back of my dad's black Lincoln Navigator. I screamed my lungs out shamelessly as my dad careered toward the hospital.

"I'm pretty sure I am dying," I moaned, gripping my stomach.

"Where does it hurt?" my dad asked, speeding over potholes, speed bumps—every barrier in his path.

"Where my heart is. It's a..." I paused, taking a deep breath in, the pain making its way through my chest. "I think it's a heart attack."

"You're not having a heart attack. When was the last time you went to the bathroom?" my mom asked, concerned but rational.

"I am having a heart attack and you are questioning my bowel movements? Ouch." I pushed my knees against my stomach and clenched hard.

"You'll be fine, just try to relax." My mom flipped her hair out of her face. Her freckles were extra prominent, standing out against her sun-kissed skin. She didn't like how they looked, but I thought they were so cute. I started counting them, a good distraction, trying not to think about the pains—*ouch*, not working!

Well, we got to the hospital, and, lucky for me, or unlucky for me: (1) it was not a heart attack, (2) my mom was right; it was constipation and dehydration from not drinking enough fluids, and (3) the volunteer EMTs at the hospital went to my high school, and I totally made eye contact with a group of them on the way in. *Awesome*. I didn't need a heart attack, because I died of embarrassment the moment we locked eyes. It ended in an enema, with me squealing like a pig. Literally, imagine, *"SQUEEEEAAAAAAAAAALLLL!!!"* I'll let you take that scene in. Yep.

So, that summer in Nantucket, my mom bought me ex-lax to prevent the Squeal Heard 'Round the World, Part II. The first time I swallowed two pills and experienced horrible stomach cramping, I was a little scared. But then it seemed like everything that was in my stomach forced its way out, and I felt lighter. What an amazing discovery: I was Christopher Columbus landing in the New World! Eating and clearing my system with just a few pills was a miraculous weight-loss strategy. How did I not know about this? I kept the bottle and used it throughout the entire vacation.

Using laxatives made me feel good. They gave me the same empty feeling that starving myself did, but I was allowed to eat and be temporarily full. It was perfect for the days when I slipped and couldn't help but binge. Yes, it was painful, but that made the crime fit the punishment. But there was a catch. I just wasn't aware of it. Yet.

I had just left a therapy session with Dr. Blatter and walked into the icy winterscape that was New York City's Upper West Side. Dr. Blatter is a quiet, medium-sized man, always well dressed in a suit and tie. His office is in a building with a green awning on Columbus Avenue and 73rd.

I had been seeing him for about five years. For most of that time, I had talked about my problems with work, lack of reliable friends, my family, things that pissed me off. I hadn't been honest about my extracurricular anorexic/not-so-sober activities because I was ashamed to tell him, or maybe afraid he would send me away or hospitalize me, because, *yes, I was hurting myself.*

I'd started seeing him after spending a long weekend in Vegas for my mom's fiftieth birthday. Observing my eating patterns, Mom made sly little comments about my eating all weekend. On the last day, she finally erupted.

I'd been pushing my food around and hardly eating anything. I'd thought I was doing a pretty good job at disguising it. Apparently not. Mom's constant meal commentary should have been a clue.

"Dani, I can't watch you do this to yourself anymore. You need help!" she'd screamed, which prompted me to run onto the Vegas Strip in hysterics. A dramatic eruption deserves a dramatic reaction. She demanded I see a therapist, and to get her off my back, I agreed.

"You know how paranoid moms are?" I'd explained to Dr. Blatter at that first session. "Especially crazy Jewish moms—it's their joy, I swear! I used to struggle with my eating, but I am fine." I knew he would understand how paranoid Jewish moms are, being a religious Jew himself—plus, it underplayed her concern, proving my point. *Nice touch, Dani.* My hands were crossed on my lap, eyes looking straight into his.

It had taken five years. Five years, countless nights of misery, and a terrifying health scare. But we were finally talking about my real problems, and as I turned the corner and hailed a cab, I knew I was on my way to *really* being fine. A driver stopped, and I hopped into the back of his cab. *Thank goodness,* I thought, as my breath had been visible in the frigid air.

"Traffic, that sucks," I said, observing the back-to-back bumper traffic around us.

"Yes, it's bad traffic tonight for some reason," the driver answered and put on the radio to some soft African music. It was pretty catchy, and I let the driver know that. He laughed, smiled, and turned the volume up a little more. I stared out the window and into the stream of traffic. The horns honking, none of it bothered me.

As I often do, I thought about the time I'd lost to my ED, short for "eating disorder," an abbreviation coined by author and eating disorder survivor Jenni Schaefer in *Life Without ED.* I was always thinking about what ED took from me because, let's face it, it took a shitload, especially the last four years of my adult life. When I was mad at my eating disorder, I was mad at myself, but recently, I'd found it helpful to separate the two in order to stop blaming myself. I had been reading *The Eating Disorder Sourcebook,* and in it, author Carolyn Costin describes two versions of yourself—your eating-disordered self and your healthy self. The idea is that your healthy self will eventually heal your eating-disordered self.

Dr. Blatter and I had just talked about that, and about what I would write if I wrote a letter to my eating-disordered self.

Dear Eating-Disordered Self,

Well, what can I say? You sure put me through the wringer. You isolated me, harmed me, made me extremely depressed, and gave me a lot of health complications. You convinced me that we were codependent. I know I could never ever be as hard on someone else as you were on me. I think that is why I am oftentimes considered too cautious of everything I say and have a bad "sorry" habit. The last thing I would ever want to do is make someone feel as bad as you made me feel. You beat me down, ruined my relationship with not only food, but also everyone, and pushed my healthy self into submissive invisibility. I am now braver, stronger, and more carefree since I defeated you. Though I may have my down days, when I hear your whispers I know I have conquered you because I used to hear you in screams. Though we have spent so much time together, I am too happy living life to ever see you again.

Best Regards,
My Healthy Full Self

I posted my letter on Facebook when I got home. Then I took my dog, Teddy, in my arms and enjoyed his butterfly kisses. I'd had Teddy, a four-pound Shih Tzu, since I was nineteen years old.

I'd named him after my love for teddy bears as a child, when I was young and innocent, and everything seemed so easy and attainable. Back then I used to go to FAO Schwarz, where I'd marvel at the big ticking clock and marching soldiers as "Welcome to my World of Toys" played its sing-song lyrics in the background. My mom and dad would let me choose one bear per visit. I would stare at the bears until my parents were blue in the face. I would always pick the one that was a little disheveled, the one whose eyes were uneven or had a crooked nose: the corduroy bear of the bunch. I wanted to help the one that was different or looked like no one else would buy it. I thought its flaws were what made it adorable—loveable even. Too bad it took me a while to feel that way about myself.

I looked back down at Teddy, a great companion, but he couldn't be my everything. Unfortunately, he couldn't fix the whole mess my eating disorder had caused; actually, he couldn't fix any of it. I needed to be my own Lisa, the girl who helped Corduroy like himself the way he was. Yes, I needed to sew my broken button back on and put the pieces of my life back together. I needed to like myself again before anyone else could. All I knew was that I was well on the way, with my healthy FULL self now running the show. This self deserved to be liked and maybe even loved.

When school started up again, I devised a plan for stocking up on laxatives. After school or during a free period, I would drive to a drugstore out of town. I'd never make a direct line to the right aisle, even though I knew exactly where the magic pills would be. Instead, I'd browse the makeup aisle, then make a right and a left in the baby aisle by accident, then over one to pretend I had a headache, until finally I got to my destination. Turn left, turn right, coast clear, and I'd grab the box, my preference at the time being the ninety-count ex-lax.

They came in handy, especially on late nights when I was the only one awake. All day I would not eat anything, thinking, *this is the day when I start my diet,* but after playing soccer for a couple of hours and starting my homework late, I needed a lot of willpower to stay up on an empty stomach. Often, I was not strong enough. One night in particular, I tiptoed into the kitchen and took a cinnamon raisin bagel, paused, and on second thought, slathered peanut butter on it. It was like an orgasm in my mouth—or at least what I imagined an orgasm to feel like. I went back to the computer room to study my notes and textbook and eat it.

Between bites and turning pages, my tired mind wandered to what had happened in AP history earlier that day. With my cramping hand, I had been transcribing everything the teacher had said. A friend had looked over at my notes and laughed out loud, signaling to the boy on the other side of me to look at something on my desk, but I still wasn't completely paying attention to my periphery, until he too broke out in laughter.

"If something is so funny, I think you should share it with the class," the teacher barked at my friend and the boy, annoyed by the interruption in his lesson plan.

"Dani just wrote down the joke you made," my friend explained through her giggles.

That was the moment I put my pencil down long enough to realize they were laughing at me. Personally, I didn't think it was *that* funny. Like, seriously, "Ha, ha, ha?" And my actions were totally explicable! I hadn't realized it was a joke because I'd been too busy writing down every word the teacher said, to read later. But of course, I wasn't going to explain this—and I wasn't going to admit my processing issue—so now the entire class had a good laugh at my expense. *Thanks, friend.*

It took a lot for me to keep up with the naturally smart kids. Now everyone knew I was dumb. I slammed the textbook closed. What was the point of trying to stick to my diet? I had already failed today. The moment I decided to eat that bagel with peanut butter sealed the failing deal. I went to the kitchen for:

Two more cinnamon raisin bagels with peanut butter *and* jelly

A wide slice of ham-and-cheese quiche

Honey-roasted peanuts (by the handful)

Raisin Bran with skim milk

And so began a new habit. Each time I studied and thought about something that had happened that day that upset me, I would eat away my anxiety. I consumed the food so fast that there was little enjoyment of the taste, but it felt so good going down. However, no sooner did it thump into the pit of my stomach than I'd feel remorse. My protruding belly was the proof of my gluttony. *I am so gross.*

And off I went to my stash of laxatives: ninety pills, one by one. It was one thing I was truly excellent at—pill-popping—a skill that I would grow to appreciate and continue to hone. It would take me less than ten minutes to get all of those blue pills down, which ironically tasted quite sweet on the outside. All night long, I'd hold my stomach in the fetal position. I'd hear noises and, at times, think something was bursting inside of me, but I deserved it—all of it. The pain, the remorse, and the hatred I had for myself. I would then erupt in a secluded bathroom downstairs, with the sink water on full blast to help mask the noises.

My mom found evidence of these binges on multiple occasions. I would hide a jar of empty peanut butter that I'd consumed the night before in a drawer in the computer room, along with wrappers and anything else I'd had to peel open. She mentioned these findings a couple of times, but I uncomfortably brushed them off. My mother would nag that I would attract mice and bugs, but she didn't understand. I didn't want to throw my evidence in the garbage. It seemed more visible in the garbage, like I had accepted that I had eaten it.

By the second half of junior year, my bingeing and purging turned into a nightly ritual. I was in denial of the effects until I was forced onto the scale at the doctor's office for a checkup: 124 pounds! *Did I see that right? Shit. I. Did.* I had managed to gain twenty-four pounds in a couple of months. This was surely a record of Guinness proportions! Why hadn't the laxatives worked? They were supposed to clean out my system. Imagine how big I would have been if I hadn't taken them. All that pain and for what? To wind up an even fatter pig. Out of shame for how I looked, I tried to think of ways to convince my parents that they *really* didn't want senior-year pictures of me, which I had to take at the end of junior year—lucky me. That didn't work. When I got them back, I looked like a large slug-like alien, maybe a cousin or sister (the resemblance was *that* uncanny) of Jabba the Hutt. Where did those two chins come from? I was horrified and ripped one of the five-by-seven pictures into tiny pieces, crying angry tears. Even my mom admitted it wasn't my best picture.

So began my crash diet. No food until dinner and only healthy steamed foods when I did eat. I wasn't going to binge anymore either. I needed to face my reality, and the truth was, I was *fat*. That night I went into my bathroom, turned the shower water on to mask what I was *really* doing, and locked the door. I stripped down to fully examine my reflection. My face had become so round and puffy. The backs of my legs had cottage-cheese cellulite on them. My stomach was slightly protruding, and I don't even want to get into how big and flabby my butt was. I held a chunk of my lardy ass in my hand.

I despised the person looking back at me. This person lacked self-control. She lacked basic discipline. I flopped onto the cold marble floor and lay there, sobbing. All I could see were the naturally skinny girls in school, the girls who didn't worry about their weight and ate whatever they wanted. I always had to be on a diet, I always had to study extra hard. The more I cried, the more I conjured more proof that not only was I fat, but I was a failure, and the whole world was in on that secret *way* before me. Like the time at the blood drive at school, when the nurse saw right through me:

Nurse in the blood truck: "How much do you weigh?"

Me: "I haven't weighed myself in a while, but I think I'm around a hundred fifteen pounds."

Nurse (scanning me from head to toe): "Oh honey, you are *way* more than that."

As my blood filled the bag, the nurse's words echoed in my head. *I must look like a monster! Why would she say that otherwise?* "You are *way* more than that." *I am so fat and ugly.* "You are *way* more than that." *I hate myself. Maybe this blood will drain out of my body, and I'll disappear. She is telling you the truth, and she is unbiased!* "You are *way* more than that." *Listen to her.*

I did it, voice, I listened good and hard.

✕

Why had I let myself get to this point? I had to pull myself together. I slowly got up off the bathroom floor and put my clothes back on. I wiped away my tears and turned the shower off. This was my fault, my doing, and I would be the one to fix it. I put my fake smile on and went downstairs to do my homework, passing my mom on the way to the computer room. She was reading a book at the kitchen table.

"How's it going?" she asked, eyes following me as I came toward her.

I gave her a kiss on the forehead and shot her a smile. "I have a lot of homework to do, but I'm good."

"Don't study too hard. Good luck."

"Thanks," I answered, shutting the door to the computer room and, at the same time, on the pathetic fat girl whose reflection stared back at me in the mirror. So long, Jabba's cousin, sister, whoever that hideous creature was looking back at me. The one I didn't recognize, and didn't *ever* want to get to know. The truth was, if I had a choice about which *Star Wars* character to resemble, I would much rather be an adorable Ewok—a skinny as fuck one.

CHAPTER 4

Denial

In my senior year, I did something really hard—I quit soccer. I know, dramatic lead-up for what it was, but it was *really* hard for my teenage self. The sport I once loved had grown to feel more like a job I resented. Plus, I didn't need to play in order to get into college, because I had worked hard to attain and maintain a 4.1 GPA. Side note: I bombed my SAT's due to my testing anxiety/refusal to take extra time for my processing problem. My Ivy League dreams were dead with my mediocre test score, flushed down the toilet with all my other failures (and food purges), but I still had my high GPA to lean on.

Soccer had been a constant in my life, an enormous part of who I was. I had begun kicking the ball around even before I started school. My elementary, middle-school, and high-school years had been dedicated to soccer summer camps, school teams, and club teams. All my life, my parents dropped everything to drive me to away games and tournaments as far as Miami. But by senior year, it seemed I didn't have the emotional and physical strength to keep up.

My high school team had nine girls in my grade, all of whom were best friends, popular girls who liked to party, and who saw me as a little study-hard goody-two-shoes and let me know it. The coach favored me, which only fueled their disdain. They made me feel like even more of an outsider than I did walking the high school halls.

I opened my mesh Nike gym bag only to discover I had forgotten my soccer cleats at home.

"Dammit!" I whispered loudly as I placed both my hands behind my head in frustration.

I decided my best bet was to speed home and grab my cleats before practice started and anyone noticed my absence. All was going according to plan until, on the way back to the field, an old man made a left turn into my car, skidding it into the side of the road. When I got back to the field I was visibly shaken, and practice had already begun.

"I am so sorry I am late," I breathed in to fight back the tears. "I got into a really scary car accident. Everyone is okay, but I am a little shaken up." I had some tears in my eyes and my voice quivered.

Behind me I saw one of the girls, Melanie, clearly mocking me as the other girls laughed. "I was in a terrible car accident. I am such a loser, poor baby me..." She went on and on, but I couldn't hear the rest of what she was saying through my coach's response.

"You shouldn't have come back. That's very dedicated, but go home and..." I couldn't focus on either conversation because I was trying to listen to both, Melanie and the coach.

My heart sank to the pit of my stomach. Now I knew it for certain—my senior teammates thought I was "such a loser."

So, even though I finished my senior-year season on the school team as captain, it was nothing like being the captain of the football team and ruling the school. In fact, being captain felt more like a curse than a blessing, and it definitely had something to do with how I came to the position.

The way my coach determined who was captain was by anonymous vote. Three girls were named captain. Unsurprisingly, I was not one of them. But having been on varsity since freshman year and being the first freshman girl in my town's history to be named "First Team All-League," I thought I deserved the title. *Here is another disappointment to add to your growing list of failures.*

I was upset but got over it, after the initial shock. My mom did not. She was *pissed*, to put it mildly. She, along with other moms on the team, called the coach and embarked on the "Dani not being captain is an injustice" crusade. After enough complaints, I was named captain number four. This most definitely added even more fuel to those nine hate fires, keeping them nice and toasty with contempt.

I had an interesting role on my high-school team. I was the center midfielder and assisting machine. I had the most assists at the end of the season every year. I was also the one to take shots during penalty kicks because of my accuracy with placement. I could trick the goalkeeper and go to the other side of the net. The problem was, on the field, I would never shoot. I preferred to give the other girls the glory, afraid I would upset them more if I drew more attention to myself. So I would make the team look good. But there was more: something inside of me didn't give me the confidence to score a goal. "Dani, shoot the ball!" screamed my coach, Mom, Dad, and the crowd.

No! Instead, I'd find the perfect assist and we would score, but I didn't want any of the praise. I wasn't worthy of it. I didn't deserve it.

As the season progressed, my speed had gotten slower from a cocktail of shin splints mixed with constant purging and dieting. Not a great combination for a soccer player.

I surrender, I surrender, I wanted to scream when my high-school season came to a close—but it wouldn't be that easy. *Without soccer, your dad will not be proud of you anymore,* screamed my inner voice. My dad was so proud of my soccer playing—it gave him "dad bragging" rights. He'd never been a student, so grades didn't impress him, but my soccer accolades did. It was our bonding time, a big part of our relationship. Without it, would he even love me anymore? *No, No, NOOO. He will not.*

I remember driving with him to a tournament in Miami during winter break; I turned to him and broke down.

"Dani, what's wrong?" he asked, taking his eyes off the road long enough to see my face all red and covered in tears.

"I just can't do it anymore. I hate it. I am so sorry," I said, hands covering my face.

"Dani, I always told you when it wasn't fun anymore you should stop," he said, glancing over at me again.

It's true; he had always reminded me of that, but it's the sort of thing I thought he was just saying because I was his daughter, like when my mom told me how "beautiful" I was.

"I feel so bad because you and Mom have done so much. I don't want to disappoint you guys," I said, hands still blockading my face.

"You are never a disappointment," my dad immediately replied, as he began looking for the next exit. "Let's go home."

This was too easy, like a *Brady Bunch* episode. *He is so disappointed, you idiot. Are you too dumb or blind to see that? He is just telling you what he thinks you want to hear.*

That made *much* more sense.

With that, he turned the car around, and I officially hung up my shin guards and cleats for good. And that was that: I was no longer a soccer player. I was...hmm. Who was I without that black-and-white ball? Even though that question was scary, it could no longer be avoided. *Yes, it could.* The blank stare that followed would involve some deep contemplation on my part. *Fill that void with hunger and you won't have to answer it yet. Numb out for a little longer.* Okay, voice, if you insist...

Now that I'd quit soccer and gotten early acceptance into Babson College, outside of Boston, I could really enjoy senior year. My first priority became losing the weight I couldn't take off during soccer season because I needed to eat to have energy on the field. *Good excuse, fat ass. Real disciplined people have all the energy in the world without food.* Second on my agenda was increasing my class rank. Focused, I began a strict food diet, along with a diet of textbooks, a far cry from the priorities my classmates had made of partying and drinking. I steered clear. Alcohol contained empty calories and losing control wasn't for me; I was the good girl.

Part of being a good girl meant staying away from boys. If I were to kiss boys, be carefree, experience pleasure, I might do something wrong. A boy's touch would make me nervous; maybe I would be tempted to be impulsive—and make a mistake. Catch-22: because I refused to do anything, I felt so inexperienced that I was afraid I wouldn't be good at engaging in the simplest romantic acts, like kissing, so my inner perfectionist was reluctant to even try.

My first kiss finally happened in my sophomore year with a guy who looked exactly like one of the Property Brothers on HGTV— no joke, he could possibly be a long-lost triplet! As I trembled to the point where I was literally holding down my leg with all my might, we kissed. As his tongue jutted into my mouth, I sweated—dripping flop sweat. I could picture Paris Hilton saying, in her signature baby voice, "That's hot," because she said that about everything, but this was anything but.

I had heard rumors about bad kissers, and I didn't want to be one of them. But I also liked my image as the good girl, and I wanted to keep it. My reputation became more important than exploring new sides of myself—parts of me that I was sure to meet by giving in to any temptations. I wanted to remain the girl who mothers wanted their sons to date. But I became the prude girl who horny high-schoolers didn't want to be with because they knew they weren't going to get any action.

At night, as my tummy would rumble, I'd grab the bottle of I Can't Believe It's Not Butter and spray the faux-buttery liquid into my mouth. Zero calories per shot. Yum. When I wanted a change, I would put Splenda in the bottle so, when I sprayed it into my mouth, there was a sweet taste. I doused everything with this magic spray, even bland steamed chicken or shrimp. When I slipped from my diet and binged, which by this point was only once a week (thanks to my motivational Jabba pictures), I'd run upstairs to the hiding spot in my closet and retrieve a suitcase filled with boxes of ex-lax, buried under clothes. I would pop the pills into my mouth, one after another, and wait for the pain, a signal that everything I had piggishly eaten was about to come out.

FULL LIFE, DECEMBER 2013

This was my last meeting as part of this Women's Associates Committee. I stormed out of it knowing I had made the right decision. I would send an email with my resignation. I'd made my decision when one of the leaders bitchily tossed her hair and laughed pretentiously while presenting how she envisioned the Spring Gala—her way being the only way. It was my final-straw moment after a series of bullying, sorority-girl-like tactics from her: dismissing others in the group, bossing people around, and treating people only in accordance with what they brought to the table socially and financially. This girl thought she was *Gossip Girl's* very own Blair Waldorf, queen bee of Constance, and we were all her little minions. After all I had been through, I sure as hell hadn't signed up to be a minion.

As a member of this nonprofit group's associates committee, I'd supported them throughout the four rock-bottom years of my eating disorder. I liked the group of girls and its initiatives, but one of the group's leaders was very controlling, creating a negative environment for all. No one else was allowed to have a voice, and if you did, this lady sure as hell didn't want to hear it. She also made it pretty clear that she wasn't a fan of me, at least, by never giving me the time of day—probably because I wore sweatpants and wasn't into the whole fashion world that ruled her day-to-day. I had invested so many years into this organization and into trying to prove myself to her that I felt attached. I'd stayed because I felt guilty—like I was in a bad relationship I couldn't break away from because I was afraid of being without it. I'd stayed too long.

I believed in the cause, but it also wasn't my main passion anymore, if I was completely honest. I also didn't want to disappoint the group by leaving. What would they think? After that final-straw moment, I left to do things that made me happier and feel more fulfilled. I think there are some important lessons learned here. The first time something you are doing has a negative impact on you, get the hell out, no matter what. Also, haters gonna hate, not everyone is going to like you—and sometimes for no reason at all. Sometimes you and that special person are just destined to be Biggie and Tupac. But you know what? I didn't care that I wasn't her cup of tea, because she wasn't my cup of tea either. In fact, she was more like a cup of coffee to me—and I don't like coffee. So that night I posted on my Living a FULL Life Facebook page:

Not one drop of my self-worth depends on your acceptance.

I have trouble with this at times. I find myself obsessing about what I should say. "Did I say it right?" I often ask after a conversation. "Was I okay?" And then if the person says, "Yes," I panic. "Just okay, not great?" Setting myself up for disaster. Never let your self-worth depend on what others think. Someone is always going to find something wrong with you if they want to. You can't be everyone's perfect person, but you can be your own person, and that is by far good enough. So please accept yourself as you are, and your self-worth will skyrocket.

Trusting my instincts, I now am happier and feel I am helping people the most by fighting for something so close to my heart—eating disorder recovery. I ended up where I was supposed to be by not people-pleasing, and by doing what truly made my heart sing. Old Dani would have tried to get the queen bee to like her, fighting until her gravestone read "Death by feet, because she was a doormat." New Dani wasn't going to waste her time. Oh, and another takeaway: when I want to get really mad, I picture that girl flipping her long brown hair and obnoxiously fake-laughing, and then I whip out my secret kung fu moves. Kidding, but maybe one day. You never know...High-Ya!

Over the last six months of senior year, the weight melted away—and I felt good about heading off to college as disciplined as I was. While people warned me about the impending "freshman fifteen," I knew I had laid the groundwork for that to never be me.

I never told anyone what I was doing, not even my mom. I knew she would try to stop me. And, no way in all that is good and holy was I going to let that happen.

"Are you okay?" asked a former math teacher in her thick Russian accent. "You look really *so* skinny." She was a tall, heavyset woman with short brown hair and a noticeable gap between her front teeth. It was hard not to stare at it, even though I tried with all my willpower not to.

"Yes, I am okay, just stressed from studying so hard for finals and APs." *Shit*, I caught myself staring at the gap again. I quickly returned my gaze to her eyes, then looked back down at her feet. I couldn't lie to her dead in the face.

But her insinuation infuriated me to the core. *Just because I lost some weight that I clearly needed to lose doesn't mean I am unhealthy.*

The truth was, I wasn't okay. My feelings of being overwhelmed, not good or smart enough, out of place, out of control, and not sure of my identity without soccer were crushing me. And starving was my only coping mechanism.

Before I knew it, it was time for senior prom. I didn't really want to go, but my friends were going, and I wanted to feel like I fit in for once. Now that I was skinnier, maybe I had a chance.

No one asked me to the prom, which was kind of expected—don't worry, no sad violins playing on my behalf—so I asked my best guy friend, Mathew, from a neighboring town. As far as attire, I decided to borrow one of my mom's slinky red Valentino dresses instead of going through the shameful torture of shopping. Don't even get me started on that pastime. With each outfit I tried on, I would see every flaw on my body, every roll, and every imperfection. Shopping served as a big self-loathing trigger and self-esteem deflator. The sizes would define me. If I were a size zero, I was doing well. If I were any size bigger...well, that would be an automatic binge/purge fiasco.

Mom letting me borrow her dress saved my sanity. Plus, she always had amazing style, an eye for fashion, and a closet with endless options. *How were we related again?* She let me alter it to my size, and I was actually okay with how it hung on my increasingly skinny frame. *Okay*, because I was never satisfied with what I saw in the mirror. I only saw something that needed improvement—a constant work in progress.

Photos were being taken at my good friend Dawn's house. I got my hair and makeup done while my mom talked and laughed with me. Then we ate lunch at my favorite sushi place, Hanami. As I looked at the menu, I started to self-consciously play with my stomach with my hands, feeling it, in anticipation of filling it.

"I only want something light. I don't want to bloat in my dress," I admitted to Mom while looking over my ordering options.

"That's insane!" Mom exclaimed but let me get away with only two pieces of tuna sashimi, despite her and the waitress's disapproval.

"She so skinny already," the waitress said to my mom. "Tiny girl," she added as she placed food and chopsticks in front of us. This reaction was a far cry from *Jabba-gate* only a couple of months back, I happily thought, smiling to myself.

"Yes, I know. She *is* being crazy," my mom said, giving me strong side-eye.

"Okay, I get the point. Look, I am eating!" I said, looking down at my two pieces of tuna sashimi and shoving one piece into my mouth. "Did you pay the waitress to say that?" I added, with slight paranoia mixed with jest.

"I don't know what I am going to do with you," my mom sighed and began eating her Hanami special roll, which consisted of two kinds of tuna, salmon, lobster salad, and avocado, wrapped in sliced cucumber. I loved that roll, but it was too much food for me these days. I watched her eat as I sipped on Diet Coke.

Later in the day, as she helped me slip the dress on, she glowed with pride. In response, I did a little spin for effect, the dress flowing in circles. "So beautiful," she marveled, and I took a bow, completing my performance. *Okay, Mom, I know you have to say that, especially at prom.* I had to be silly to get through the moment, the attention, all of it. I thanked her and smiled. Even with makeup painted on my face and my hair done stick straight, I didn't feel anything near beautiful.

My dad came home from work early that day, and tears filled his dark brown eyes when he saw me. His little girl, who he had cradled not too long ago—in his mind at least—was going to prom.

"Who is this woman? And where is my little girl?" he said.

"Oh my goodness, Dad, no more! I hate this kind of attention, but I love you," I said, wanting to off myself with embarrassment.

"Learn to take a compliment. You look beautiful."

"No more! Thank you!" I screamed, holding my ears in protest, as we headed to the car.

The time came to head out for prom pictures. As we pulled up, I shivered with social anxiety, as I could smell the strong odor of teen angst in the air.

As we entered Dawn's house, I gave my friends hugs and cheek kisses and told them how beautiful they looked, as I looked around for Mathew. There were appetizers spread around the house and drinks for the parents (and sneaky kids who would take a couple of sips when their parents weren't looking or turned a blind eye). But I didn't want to look at the food or chance anyone offering me anything I would have to decline.

There he was: Mathew, dolled up in a tuxedo, like my very own penguin. I was *so* happy to see him, my comfort in the prom chaos.

"Hi there, you stud," I joked as I gave him a big bear hug. "I like this whole penguin look; it suits you well." I paused. "Or, should I say, *tuxedos* you well."

"Your jokes suck, Dani." He smiled back at me.

"You look handsome. You get the point!" I said laughing.

"Handsome like a penguin, I'll take that."

"Picture time!" shouted one of the mothers. "Everyone get together!"

"Perfect timing. We wouldn't want to miss pictures. I mean, heaven forbid." I winked at my date, placing my hand jokingly over my mouth, as we moved to the backyard.

Between the camera flashes that briefly blinded me, I could tell Dawn's mother was looking at me peculiarly, and I started fidgeting in response. I rubbed my cheeks; did I have a makeup smudge? Even so, she didn't have to stare and make me feel more insecure and out of place than I already did.

As I was walking around after pictures, looking for my parents, she approached. "Hi, Dani. You look beautiful, but…I think you are losing too much weight. You're so frail." She grasped my arms and looked at me like she was reading me my last rites—*so dramatic.*

"I am fine, I promise, but thanks," I said, taking her hands off my body and backing a few steps away. Like two cowgirls in the Wild West, we stared at each other, in a standoff of sorts. It appeared she had nothing else to say and neither did I, so I unloaded my lipstick for touch-ups and walked away pretending it was time to reapply. Hopefully, this interaction would never be spoken of again.

How dare she judge me! I don't look too thin. Why did she have to point me out as different and ruin the night before it even started? I am not bingeing as much as I was, so I am actually healthier and she has no idea what she is talking about. Clearly.

Looking back, it's like I was becoming a politician, accomplished in denial.

But Dawn's mom's reaction also felt ironic to me. When I was Jabba-the-Hutt fat and making myself sick with laxatives every night, no one said anything, but now that I was skinny, *that* was considered unhealthy and a cause for concern? I didn't really get it. Alanis Morissette would understand me on this, because, yeah, it really was a little too ironic, don't you think?

I found my mom, venting to her about what had happened with Dawn's mom. The nerve of her, right? How dare she! I was visibly upset, fuming from her rude and poorly timed comments. "Don't listen to that, sweetheart," she counseled. "Dawn's mom didn't choose the right time to say something, that's all."

The right time? What did my mom mean by that?

She thinks you are a freak like everyone else. Thanks for the prompt answer, voice.

The night was okay overall. After the dance, all of the seniors went to a club rented by a popular boy in our grade. I didn't drink and tolerated drunken friends stumbling and clinging to me, blabbering, "Dani, I LOVE you, like, so much."

"Thanks." I would smile and laugh a little to myself. Why did high-school kids have to always get so sloppy drunk? And, come on, I knew half of them were exaggerating the effects to seem cool. My parents and their friends never got like this when they drank. Well, actually, I take that back. Maybe once in a while, but they certainly didn't act like these idiots. Maybe I just needed to start drinking so I could be a carefree kid too. Who really knows? The only thing I knew at that moment was that intoxicated high schoolers liked me a lot better than sober ones, and right now it was working in my favor.

"Dani, I think you look very prettyyyyy," said Mathew. He draped his arm over my back, trying to be slick through his slurred English.

"That's because you are a little intoxicated, buddy," I said, removing his arm and looking at my watch. *Get me out of here!*

He insisted that I drive him home last, and right when he was getting out of the car, he leaned in to kiss me. As his lips closed in on my face, I panicked, turning fast and giving him an accidental cheek. He was just my good friend, and I didn't want to ruin it. Also, even if I did like him a little more than a friend, he was wasted and I was sober. Why would I kiss someone completely shit-faced? Exactly, I wouldn't, unless I was shitfaced too, of course. I have values, come on.

I felt terrible on my drive home. It wasn't just the kiss, it was that damn skinny comment playing on repeat in my head. *Too skinny. Frail.* I shook my head from side to side, gripping the wheel. No, I didn't have a problem. I was in total control of this. I was *so* responsible. I knew what I was doing. Look at these damn drunken delinquents; they were clearly the ones with issues! Come on! Right? Right...

I couldn't lie to my subconscious. Deep down, I knew I was the messed-up one. I really wished I could be one of those carefree normal teenagers, but I didn't have it in me. And now that I realized that people were taking notice, all I knew for certain, besides that I couldn't wait to get into bed and close my weary eyes, was that I was ready to get the hell out of this small town.

I was in Miami on vacation with my family for the long weekend. It was the Chinese New Year and we went to Christine Lee's, an all-time Sherman favorite Chinese restaurant. It was a hot and humid night, leaving my hair frizzing in all directions. I'd patted it down with gel before we left, but it had plans of its own. We had a big family-style meal, with all sorts of food. I stuck with mu shu chicken and egg drop soup and sipped on a Grey Goose on the rocks to wash it all down. While our table was being cleared, people dressed up as dragons appeared, seemingly out of thin air, banging on gongs.

"Shit, that's so loud," I said covering my ears and screaming across the table. My mom pointed to her ear indicating that she could not hear me. "Point made!" I screamed back.

"What?" my mom screamed.

I just shook my head, *never mind*.

The gongs and loud music continued into a synchronized dance in the middle of the restaurant. People cheered from their tables. We had been going to this restaurant since I was a little girl. My grandpa used to take us when it was in a dingy strip mall. Now it was a huge restaurant in the middle of a racetrack, with fancy decorations and a huge bar. Huge bar equals my kind of place.

The music came together for the big finale, then finally silence. I applauded, a little for the performance, but more because I was so happy those loud sounds were finished.

Fortune cookies came to the table. I always loved them, because I somewhat believed them in a wanting-to-see-through-the-lens-of-a-child way, but at least I always had fun with them. I removed the cookie from the little plastic bag and cracked it open, revealing my fortune.

"Ooooh, I like this one," I said, looking up at my mom and dad.

"Let's hear it," said my dad.

"One must dare to be himself however frightening or strange that self may prove to be."

"I like that one," my mom agreed.

Later when we returned to our hotel, I decided to write a post on my Living a FULL Life Facebook page:

Just for the record I am not fortune cookie obsessed, contrary to what this FB page may portray. I know they are manufactured crisp cookies with a piece of paper, but some of them are wěidà—

Chinese for great ;) I got a wĕidà one tonight that I needed to share.
It said, "One must dare to be himself/herself however frightening
or strange that self may prove to be." I added the "herself"
because, come on, manufacturers, women have to be our strange
frightening selves too!

Embrace that inner "weird" and wear it proudly. That is the most
admirable thing a person can do, and I bet you it is not as offbeat
as you think; you are definitely not alone. Once you do own it, it
will no longer be quite as frightening to be your authentic self.
Happy Sunday <3

As I posted, my mom walked into my attached room to say
goodnight. "What was your fortune?" I asked.

Teddy was at the end of the bed, curled in a little ball,
already fast asleep.

"Help, I'm a prisoner in a Chinese fortune cookie factory,"
she said, completely straight-faced.

"Seriously?" I asked, bursting out in laughter, throwing my
wild hair back onto the soft pillow behind me.

"No, but it sounded good, right?" she said laughing.

"It sure did," I said, pulling the blanket over my chest.

"Well goodnight, Babyface," she said and gave me a kiss on
my forehead.

"Goodnight, Mommyface, I love you," I said as she shut the
door to my room.

CHAPTER 5

The Mid-Freshman-Year Crisis

My parents made the five-hour journey to Boston with me to help set up my dorm at Babson College. As they unpacked each tchotchke and memento, the pit in my stomach grew larger. When the other students were having tearful goodbyes with their parents, I did as well—please, I was a hysterical mess—but, on top of that, I worried about how I would quit my dependence on laxatives cold turkey. Now that I had a roommate and would be sharing a bathroom with many strangers, how would I get any privacy at all if I binged? I decided I would just be extra good at dieting—I'd fine-tune my expert starving skills. It was time for me to get off laxatives anyway, because bingeing was counterproductive to my weight loss. This would be easy...or maybe easier said than done.

I had my tricks to ignore the hunger pangs and make sure nobody noticed I wasn't eating: (1) Avoid social meals, explaining to people that I'd already eaten or grabbed a snack at the library. (2) When I was hungry during the day, satiate myself with gumballs, tea, and diet soda. Bottles of Diet Coke and several cups of tea with at least five packages of Splenda helped curb my appetite and appease my sweet tooth. The barista at the student center nicknamed me Earl Grey because I ordered so much of it. (3) Night food—one small bag of Rold Gold Honey Wheat Braided Pretzel Twists, total food consumption for the day.

To get as much mileage out of each pretzel as possible, I would suck the tip slowly until it was nice and soggy and then bite the top off and swoosh it in my mouth. Instead of swallowing it, I spat it out onto the other end of the pretzel to conserve it, and then I slowly proceeded to put the whole pretzel into my mouth. Chewing slowly, I'd stop before my reflex to swallow kicked in, and I'd swoosh the crumbs in my mouth for a while, spreading the salty taste before finally allowing it down my throat.

My rule was to wait ten minutes between each pretzel. But often I'd break my own ritual because I was so hungry. That tiny bag of pretzels soon became my one and only pleasure in the day. I'd wait for it, like people wait for a hot date or a glass of wine at the end of a long workweek. All day long, I'd pine for that bag, my reward for working so hard.

When my roommate was asleep, I'd reach under the covers for my bottle of I Can't Believe It's Not Butter spray, rolling away from her to spray it into my mouth, pumping as slowly as I could to mute the spritzing sound. My reward for making it through another day, showing my hunger who was *really* boss. *I was!* I could take it.

I could feel my pants getting bigger. Now I had to wear my size-twenty-six jeans with a belt at its smallest hole. I couldn't help but admire my nice flat tummy and be impressed with my discipline. Unfortunately, I couldn't starve myself forever; I was bound to slip, and that meant a purge.

It was a Friday night, a month and a half into my laxative sobriety, and I was really stressed out. I was struggling with an extremely difficult school project that was due on Monday. I had been working on it all day, but felt like I hadn't gotten anywhere. *I am going to fail. How am I going to get this done? I am so stupid.* So overwhelmed, to the umpteenth degree, I finally couldn't take it anymore. With the pressure to make progress, combined with that empty feeling taunting me from the pit of my stomach, all I could think about was food to distract me. *Fuck it all. I am a failure.* I grabbed my keys and drove to a supermarket in the town of Wellesley, five minutes from campus. Charging into the store, I manically grabbed a jar of peanut butter and a big bag of pretzels along with a loaf of whole-wheat bread and a ninety-count box of ex-lax. Why healthy whole-wheat bread would matter at that point is a mystery, but it made me feel better about what I was about to do.

I sat in my car in the parking lot eating all of it—stuffing it down my throat in chunks and pieces. Midway through eating, I took the laxatives as my punishment. Then I ate and ate, feeling my waist expanding. I shoveled the food into my mouth without taking a breath, so quickly that I could hardly taste it, but it wasn't about the taste. No matter how much I ate, I never seemed to fill that empty pit in my stomach. Tears dripped from my eyes as the nausea from the laxatives and food set in. I looked in the rearview mirror; my dark brown eyes were bright red from my rubbing them, and I had peanut butter smears around my mouth. My palms were stained with the melted blue coating of the handfuls of laxatives I'd popped into my mouth. *What was I doing?*

Suddenly overcome with the sharp contractions of my intestinal walls, I reversed the car, headed back to campus, and sprinted to the communal bathroom on my floor. I was going to be sick. As I ran past a girl taking off her makeup after a long night of drinking, I avoided eye contact, hoping she wouldn't get a good look at me. Stomach gurgling, I lurched into a corner stall with the sudden horrifying realization that she was going to hear me. I heard her giggling at my prominent stomach noises—loud hollow noises followed by embarrassingly loud gas. I was mortified, but maybe I deserved to be laughed at. Maybe the laughter would serve as a reminder to make me think twice next time I even contemplated bingeing.

I heard her exit that bathroom fast, probably to gossip to her friends about what she'd just heard and witnessed or to avoid being rude by laughing even louder. I flushed the toilet and wobbled out of the stall. Sometimes, after these binges, my equilibrium felt off, like I was coming back down to earth (after visiting some faraway galaxy, preferably Endor due to the Ewok population, but probably more like Purge-a-tory, the planet of purging) and my body couldn't adjust properly. I leaned over the sink, washing my hands with soap and water. As the water ran, I looked in the mirror. I still had a peanut butter mustache. *My reality was as pathetic as that peanut butter mustache.*

Bingeing was often spur of the moment, and there was no time to talk myself out of it before it was happening. It was like I was a remote-controlled car steered by some invisible hand. Then the reality would set in, the horrible reality—the regret, guilt, and self-loathing. I would just have to find a bathroom that was more private and plan my binges in advance. At least, if I thought about bingeing, I'd have to make sure it was a good time, where people weren't around and have the diuretics and food in stock. I had that much self-control. Hopefully.

The graduate school offered a safe spot for planned binges because it closed around eight in the evening for anyone entering, but if you were already there, you could stay as long as you wanted. As everyone left, I would take the laxatives in my private corner and get sick in what became my private bathroom. Then I would stay, studying, until two or three in the morning. When the diarrhea, accompanied by drooping, baggy, crusty eyes, was over or significantly easing up, I would drag myself across campus to my dorm, body aching and stomach sore. I'd fall helplessly into my bed, the blanket comforting my exhausted body.

Parents' Weekend was my first unplanned slip since my sticky-blue-peanut-butter-fingers incident. I was so ravenous and out of control after bingeing on Chinese food at my parents' hotel room, I couldn't stop: lo mien, chicken fried rice, sesame chicken, and fortune cookies (why do they put so many in takeout orders? Ugh). When I got back to my dorm, I did something I was not proud of. I raided my roommate's food supply and ate *her* food. I even dug through her trash to see if she'd left anything behind: a half-eaten Snickers bar—*score*. I had a bag of Cheez Doodles, peanut butter crackers, and animal crackers—anything I could get my hands on. I felt like a dirty rat, digging through the garbage. Correction, I *was* a dirty rat, digging through the garbage. Luckily for me, my roommate didn't walk in.

Shortly afterward, I hit an even lower low, losing control in front of my parents one weekend at home. They didn't see my purge, but they had noticed the copious amounts of sushi I'd put in my mouth.

"I am starving, and I don't have time to eat a lot at school because I am always studying." It was my way of saying, *Look, I eat. I am fine! My skinny body is from stress. That's all...*

I binged on every single sushi roll I could get my hands on, tempura-fried and all, a Kamikaze roll, which was perfect because I felt like a Kamikaze, so out of control and borderline suicidal in my eating patterns. Screw chopsticks, I was picking the rolls up with my bare hands and stuffing them into my mouth. I took laxatives immediately after, in the privacy of my bedroom, and was sick to my stomach all night. The next day, on the way to the shuttle back to Boston, I was burping up a rotten-egg sulfur smell in "burp-hiccups" so strong that my dad and I both gagged on the smell as he drove me to the airport. I had never smelled anything so disgusting. It was like I was burping up Newark, New Jersey, and anyone who has smelled the air in that city is familiar with the potent rotten-egg stench equivalent to an egg salad sandwich five days old. Holy "Jersey Stink!"

I can't describe how horrible that plane ride back to school was, me sweating and burping, on the verge of throwing up. On top of that, there was terrible turbulence, which made me sweat even more with anxiety. This poor Asian businessman who had the misfortune of sitting next to me, bless his soul. I will never forget his face, a look of terror mixed with awe at the smells emanating from the tiny girl beside him. By the time I made it back to school, I'd ensured my first and only absence from class, because I couldn't leave the bed. I mean, I'd just taken the entire Jersey stink to Boston, not a small feat!

I had lost even more weight, and even I knew it. By the end of the first semester, all my clothes were hanging off me. When I got dressed up to go out at night on the weekends, I would layer my outfits so no one would notice. At school, during the day, I would wear bulky sweats and sweatshirts. I once carelessly didn't layer, only wearing spandex and a Babson T-shirt to class, sweatshirt tied tightly around my waist, and one of my guy friends came over to me.

"I am worried about you. You're disappearing." He touched my frail arm, his expression turning stony-faced. I didn't even know he could get that serious. We weren't friends who had deep conversations, so I was quite taken aback.

"What do you mean? You just can't handle my guns. These babies are weapons of mass destruction," I said, while nervously laughing it off, and touched his arm back, pinching into muscle.

He laughed. "Yes, I should call the police, you are a danger to society."

"I have gotten that before. Better put this bad boy on to cover them up before someone gets hurt." I grabbed my sweatshirt and put it back on to avoid any other possible encounters like this. I'd rather be overheated than do this dance around the eating-disorder issue again—nuh-uh!

This was during finals, and I was so focused on my routines, there was no time to even look in the mirror or analyze what was happening to my body. I had to do well in all my classes or risk being even more of a failure, because it was bound to be revealed that I wasn't as smart as everyone else at college. I wouldn't let that happen.

It wasn't as easy to fool my parents as my peers. Though, let's be real, I probably wasn't fooling *anyone* with my shrinking frame. My friends just weren't going to say anything. I didn't let any of them get *that* close to me. That was my purpose in spending a lot of time alone—to avoid anyone observing my weird behaviors around food and to avoid any form of connection that could bring about a confrontation from a concerned member of the student body about my dwindling (student) body. But my parents, that was a whole 'nother story.

During winter break, my mom found a suitcase filled to the brim with empty laxative boxes. I had left the suitcase in the computer room, in a corner, thinking it was inconspicuous and no one would open it. Not my smartest move.

"Dani! What the hell are all of these?" I heard in loud, piercing echoes, the same tone she'd used back in middle and high school when I carelessly left my dirty socks everywhere, forgetting to toss them into the laundry: a sock on the kitchen chair, another sock on the table, a sock hiding in the crack of the living room couch. The list of places went on and on, and it drove my mom completely bananas—more like BANANAS! I'd hear her yells echoing through the vents, "DANI!" and that was code for "Get your butt down here now OR ELSE." Nothing made my mom more pissed-off. Except for this.

"Whoa, all of what?" I replied, startled by the tone of her voice.

"This, this..." she screamed, and shoved the now-empty black suitcase in my face, indicating that she'd found my stash—as if it weren't obvious *enough*.

"Dani, if you don't stop doing this to yourself, I..." She could hardly breathe, "I can't send you back to college."

"Mom, I am so sorry. I really will stop. I just messed up, and all of those were from a really long time of collecting, not just since I got home." Which was a lie, I'd been bingeing and purging every day since I got home.

My mom's therapist at the time, who she made me talk to after uncovering my laxative stash, was convinced I had done this subconsciously to get caught. She was totally wrong. I just had a careless moment, but I went with that because I could twist it into a good excuse for why I would never do it again. *I wanted you to catch me, Mom. Yeah right! Psh!* I would not use laxatives anymore, I reassured her. It was time for me to put an end to this anyway. I really would never touch them, I was so sorry. I wanted to believe I could do this. I wanted to believe I could stop, that I wasn't lying to her *again*. That it was truly *that* easy. These promises and discussions lasted until I went back to school for my second semester, where all I could think about was purging again.

FULL LIFE, OCTOBER 2014

Approaching the National Eating Disorders Association (NEDA) Walk, my mom and dad held hands as I trailed after them, taking in the view of all the people in green and blue NEDA shirts huddled together to keep warm. We were by the Brooklyn Bridge at Foley Square, way downtown. This was the first year I had raised money for the event. Though my team was small in numbers, it was big in pride. As I got closer to the crowd, I couldn't believe the sea of people whose lives had been touched in one way or another by this disease. For someone who always thought she was the only person in the world battling her anorexia and bulimia, this was an awe-inspiring moment.

A tall woman with kinky black hair and dark skin came to the podium and started talking about her battle with exercise bulimia and how she used to run the Brooklyn Bridge rain or shine when she attended NYU. She said she had been in recovery for six years. I remember thinking *Wow* at the notion that someone could be in recovery for that long and still be okay, and even more crazy was the fact that she was now able to fight for others, so they could see recovery is possible.

How beautiful. My dad couldn't take his eyes off this speaker; his unblinking eyes released fat tears that rolled along the contour of his chin and down his neck. He never understood people talking about their issues. He grew up in a house with an old-school mentality of being quiet about one's problems. You dealt with them, and that was it.

As we walked across the bridge, my father held my hand. "I never understood why you decided to be so public about what you went through," he told me, "but now I get it." Then he squeezed my hand, as if giving me some kind of approval.

"Thanks, Dad. I want to be able to at least help people with it. I mean, if *I* survived..." As I said that, we saw a swarm of people pass us with shirts bearing a picture of a beautiful woman that said, "In Memory of."

"Well, you help me every day," my dad said.

"Don't cry again!" I pleaded. "I am good," I said, taking my hand out of his and putting it around his back to comfort him.

"You better be," my mom interjected from behind us. She was bundled in her winter coat, lips chattering. The freezing extra-strong winds combined with the low temperatures turned her breath into mist.

As we continued across the bridge, I felt a sense of safety and solidarity. All of these people understood what I had been through—and still go through at times. I knew at that moment I would never feel alone again.

That night I posted on my Living a FULL Life Facebook page:

"Fairy tales are more than true—not because they tell us dragons exist, but because they tell us dragons can be beaten."

—G. K. Chesterton

And they can. <3

I smiled and sat back. What a great day.

Back at my dorm, I thought about how my second semester would need to be about making some much-needed changes. With my only focuses being my waistline and getting good grades, college had been kind of a bore so far. Though it was predictable and controlled, the way I liked it, I found myself disappointed with the experience. It needed a reboot of sorts, College 2.0—this version much more exciting, boozier and wilder or at least an R movie rating, I'd even settle for PG13. I didn't know it yet, but some things were about to happen that would shake me up, whether I welcomed it or not.

Change one: I became interested in not just crushing from afar but having an actual, real-life boyfriend.

I had a mini-crush on a boy at Babson and an even greater infatuation with a boy named Blake who went to New York University. He was a tall, dark, handsome, half-Filipino, and originally from my hometown. We were acquaintances who'd shared a lot of classes, the same honors path, but nothing more.

Then we found ourselves on spring break together in the Bahamas senior year of high school. We would sit and talk for hours, laughing and observing while everyone else was enjoying foam parties and the drinking age of eighteen. We were enjoying these benefits too, but in our own kind of nerdy way.

"You know what I keep thinking? That foam must be laced with vomit, beer, and..."

"Soap and water," he interrupted. We were sitting on the balcony of a club overlooking a foam-filled mosh-pit dance floor.

"Yes, but that's too obvious...more like lost room keys, spit, maybe a shirt or two," I mused, watching dancers bump their bodies against each other.

"You think people lost their tops in the foam?"

"Hell yeah, and probably on purpose. Look at them! Clearly, we aren't having enough fun! Okay, Blakey, we need to step up our game. Think I am going to go into the foam."

"I am not rescuing you, and you may get pregnant by contact."

"Good point. Then I'd have to go on *Maury* to find out who the father was, and there are too many guys here to ever know."

"You better stay here then," he laughed pulling me to his side.

"If I must," I joked, picking up my drink.

He smirked, clinking his beer with my Diet Coke. "Cheers. Spring break, baby."

"To spring break." I clinked my soda back.

Blake became one of my closest friends on this rite-of-passage trip. When we were stressed at school, we'd dream about going to a deserted island together to get away from it all. I was more comfortable being my silly self with him than I'd felt with anyone outside of family. I started to really like him, and really trust him, listening for that door-opening sound (oh yes, nineties kids, you know what I am talking about) indicating that he'd signed onto AIM (AOL Instant Messenger) so we could talk. It was like I was already in a relationship, without the physical aspect. But, I kind of wanted the physical aspect too. Who can blame a girl?

I visited Blake at school a couple of times in the first semester, once over my winter break, and though we snuggled all night in the same bed, he didn't even try to make a move. This was a little confusing. I wanted to be more than his teddy bear.

Back at school in January, I finally started drinking, wanting to have a little more excitement and feeling I was ready to try it on my own terms. I never drank beer, only vodka, which meant I could get drunk with far fewer calories. One night, during a vodka-fueled phone call, I told Blake how I felt.

"I think we should be more than friends," I blurted into my cell phone.

Silence for what seemed like a full minute.

"Okay, shit. Not a good sign." *And oh shit, I said that out loud.* In that moment, I wished I could go back in time, *Back to the Future*-style. Where was Dr. Emmett Brown when I needed him?

"I don't want to lose our friendship, Dani," he said, concluding our humiliating conversation before it had even really begun.

With my already feeble ego bruised, plus knowing I couldn't really like anyone else if I kept talking to him, I made the decision to cut off our friendship.

A week into this "friendship break," I decided to tell my other crush how I felt about him. I had heard of a midlife crisis, where the person will purchase a luxury car or undergo some expensive plastic surgery procedure. I was having a mid-freshman-year crisis and was trying to fill the void I felt with a guy. I might have been better off with an expensive car or a nose job!

We were sitting and talking outside our dormitory when I said, "I really like you," like a second-grader. But what's the right way to go about these things? Okay, maybe any way but this way...

"Well, I really like you too. You are one of my best friends here," he said, taking a sip of some strong alcohol concoction from his red Dixie cup. *Best friend*, not again, I didn't like where this was headed. I could tell.

We sat there silent. "Dani, I never had a best friend who was a girl and I really value your friendship." He briefly paused. "I don't want to lose it."

"Yeah, I totally get it." I pretended I was okay with the whole notion of being the best friend again. He gave me a hug as I fake-yawned, probably too wide, looking like I had a face spasm.

"Well, I am off to bed. I think I drank too much, and you know me. Got to be at the library early in the morning. That drink was strong." I pointed to his red Dixie cup, as his Dixie cup was a brother, made with the same alcohol, of mine.

"Yes, very strong. I hope we are okay."

"Of course we are," I said, giving him the best toothy smile I could produce, probably resembling a face spasm once again. Turning to leave, that's when my eyes started getting teary. Rejection hurts, and boy was I tired of being the good girl stuck in the friend zone.

Two weeks into our break, Blake called and said he missed me and wanted to visit me in Boston. I took that as him possibly realizing he wanted more too. To make sure of it, I pulled out all the stops. I got my hair blown out and a new fresh cut. I wanted to look really good when he arrived. I wanted him not to recognize me, but in a *who-is-that-hot-thing-sex-kitten* way. I wanted to be more than his cute and cuddly teddy bear, dammit! I wore skintight jeans that made my legs look long and booty perkier, and heels to give me some height. I could tell by how my pants fit that I had already lost the little bit of weight I'd gained over winter break, plus some since he'd last seen me. I felt a little more confident as I stood for my last look at this person in the mirror, my hardest critic, me. "You got this," I said, trying to ease my anxiety.

When he arrived, I picked him up at the train. I saw him tugging a suitcase behind him, wearing a black beanie and peacoat, kind of like Paddington Bear, but way more handsome. I parked the car and got out to help him with his bag. First thing he did, besides embracing me, was put his hand around my right wrist. "You are so tiny, Dani. What happened?" Not the reaction I was going for at all, but maybe I could rebound.

The rest of the weekend was filled with picking at food, laughing, drinking, and then our first kiss. The last night of his stay, I took him to a frat party with a bunch of my college guy friends and got the "powerful" screwdriver, which contained God knows what, to impress him. This resulted in Blake holding my hair as I hurled into the toilet, praying for my life. Not quite what I was going for, either. Alas, this was intimacy with my very first boyfriend.

✕

Change two: Elizabeth and I lost contact. She had cried and so had I when we'd headed for our respective schools. We both knew we were really leaving and growing up. Though we promised to talk all the time, I never heard from her, despite my many messages to her "Hi, this is Elizabeth, leave a message or don't bother. Peace out" recording. Eventually I gave up.

When I heard from my parents—they were very friendly with Elizabeth's—that Elizabeth had come home from college mid-semester, I was saddened. I would later hear that her friends speculated it was drugs. I could picture her dancing at a house party, the DJ (a.k.a. frat pledge) booming loud music in the background, drink in her hand, cigarette between her lips, brown hair wild, and dripping with sweat. My need to fix things and make everything perfect kicked into high gear. I wanted to go home and help take care of her, apologize for losing touch and giving up, for being a bad friend. But she needed time alone with her parents to regroup, recharge, and rehabilitate.

During March break, I went to visit her.

"Hi, I was so worried about you. I left you messages, did you get them?" I said pulling her into a warm hug. She hugged me back, but something felt different, cold and uninviting.

"Yes, but you know how college gets. I joined a sorority too, you probably heard from your parents, and it takes up a lot of my time. I am going to have a cigarette, want one?"

"No thanks, I am good." I watched her turn around and go outside, leaving me alone in her family kitchen—a place where I had spent many afternoons with Lizzie and her mom, eating snacks while doing homework. A place that felt not the same as it once had. I looked out the window, spotting Lizzie lighting her cigarette. It felt like she was over seeing me already. Had I become that obligatory friend I always feared I would be to her? Her cigarette was making wisps of silver and gray smoke dance, forming small clouds in the air above her. She was texting vigorously on her cell phone between puffs, then she dialed out, placed the phone on her ear, and walked away chitchatting. I heard her scream into the phone, "OMG! No way."

Staring at her from the side as she walked, I noticed her body for the first time. She'd lost a lot of weight, and her hair hung lank on her face. She was my polar opposite, yet here we both were wasting away, in our own unique ways. We were both changing, but I feared not for the better.

✕

Change three of this semester, or maybe I should call this strike three, was people discovering, like at camp, that something was not right with Dani Sherman. Our big end-of-semester project for my management class was to "open a business" with thirty other team members. I was responsible for the PowerPoint presentation, which in hindsight was a terrible idea, since I am not as tech-savvy as I should be. I taught myself how to navigate the program, my nerves taut as a ball of twine, but what put my anxiety over the edge was the fact that my professor didn't seem to like me. I am intuitive—I can read people extremely well—and our one-on-one conversations were awkward at best. He wasn't the kind of teacher that liked giving extra help or liked us grade-conscious folk. He liked the kids in our class who were confident, participated, and were naturally smart. I was shy and afraid to raise my hand, and because I wasn't a natural-born leader in his eyes, he didn't give me the time of day. I had never had a teacher dislike me or at least make me feel like I was a bother, and I just didn't know how to process it. I spent most of my semester kowtowing and tiptoeing and working tirelessly to prove myself to him—even participating more, which was hard for my introverted self.

The night before our nine o'clock presentation, I decided not to sleep in order to perfect my part. I tried my best but woke up in a pile of drool, draped over my books, at eight-thirty. *Shit!* Just half an hour to get across campus and begin presenting! I threw on anything I could find, hoping it would pass as "business casual," and twisted my hair into a messy bun. In my fastest soccer sprint, my computer across my body, I charged through the snow.

Out of breath, I staggered into the corridor of the building with just one minute till go-time. Well-dressed, calm, and collected, my team stared at me as I peeled my jacket off my sweaty body. I had everything ready, I assured them with a nod. I was going to be fine. I got ready to present by setting up the computer in front of the room. *Yes, I was going to be just fine...*

What seemed like a second later, the CEO of my team began to speak—my cue to begin clicking through the PowerPoint. *Be composed, you're breathing too loud, boy, it's hot in here...*

I could feel my professor's eyes burning a hole through my skin. *Focus on the presentation, Dani.* As I looked up to meet his fire eyes, I heard a buzzing in my ears and my vision fuzzed, the whole room turning blurry. *Not now, please don't faint, please.* If I sat down,

64

the professor would hate me even more. He'd be right about me, that I couldn't handle the pressure. *Just breathe, Dani.*

My mind ricocheted to fourth-grade picture day: Mom catches me in the shower after I pass out from the hot humid steam. I'm instructed by the doctor to get up slowly in the mornings and dangle my legs to get my blood flowing. I hear the faint whisper of my mom singing the song she made up to remind me to stop before I got out of bed:

> *It's time to dingle dangle dingle*
> *It's time to dingle dangle dingle*
> *It's time to dingle dangle dingle*
> *Dingle dangle time.*

I laugh as I swing my legs off the bed, up and down. Then, I smell my mom cooking my favorite breakfast, eggs over easy on an Eggo waffle...

"Danielle, Danielle, are you okay?" I heard a faraway voice. My eyes slowly opened. It was my professor, wearing a black French beret, staring down at me, concerned. It was rumored that he'd had a severe heart attack over winter break, and, ever since, he'd worn that flat-crowned hat in different colors. Every. Single. Day. His weird version of a midlife crisis? Perhaps.

At that moment, I realized, *shit,* I was on the floor and, *ouch,* with a terrible splitting headache. "Please go on with the presentation," I gushed, and I heard a roar of nervous laughter from my classmates. "I am so sorry," I gasped to my professor as he helped me sit up.

I would later learn that my eyes had rolled to the back of my head (think *The Exorcist*), as I'd fallen backward, slammed into the chalkboard, and then flopped to the floor.

Even though I had insisted on continuing with the presentation, my professor was understandably nervous because I had hit my head on that damn blackboard, so he called an ambulance and excused me from class. When they arrived, I convinced the EMTs and paramedics that I was okay and didn't need a hospital, and since I was over eighteen, they didn't force me to go. I was left in the hallway outside the classroom, humiliated and ashamed.

I told Blake the whole sordid tale. "And then I opened my eyes and thought I was in hell. My professor was hovering above me like he was about to perform CPR. What did I do to deserve this? Mouth to mouth with Meanie-Professor-Fire-Eyes? I'd have to bleach my whole mouth." Blake was on the other end, laughing. I explained it was because I had terrible anxiety, which was true, and I wanted to believe that was the only reason I'd fainted.

My mom, on the other hand, immediately began catastrophizing. "Dani, do you need me to come to campus?"

"God, no! I'm fine, I promise. You know how much anxiety I have."

"Yes, I know," said my mom, "but I'm worried about you." I could hear the concern growing in her voice.

"I promise, Mom, I am going to get tea and a bagel, and then I will take a nap."

"Okay, promise me that." This was my mom's last request before she hung up. I hung on to those last words. *Promise me that.*

What I didn't tell her was that I hadn't eaten a real meal in weeks. *Promise me that.* I didn't tell her that my pants were big in the waist and thighs, which I admired tirelessly in the mirror. *Promise me that.* I also failed to mention that my eyes had permanent bags and my skin was pale white like a clown's painted face. *Promise me that.* Oh yeah, and worst of all, I still used laxatives, even though I'd sworn I wouldn't. *Promise me that.* I clearly couldn't.

I returned to my dorm after that conversation and changed into my workout clothes. *A workout will make you feel better. Lessen the shame.* I then spent an hour on the elliptical machine, sweat pouring from every inch of my body, just the way I liked it. Endorphins giving me the temporary high I so badly needed.

FULL LIFE, JANUARY 2014

"What are you doing?" my mom asked, peering into the living room. I was hanging with Teddy at my parents' house for the day. "I am trying to get into my mindset during my sick times," I said, without thinking.

"That's a little scary, Dan," my mom said, sitting next to me on the big comfy tan couch.

"Just for Mental Health Awareness Day, for a post," I reassured her. "I'm fine."

"Okay." She grimaced at Teddy, as if he would agree with her reticence. I don't think she wanted me to go back to that place for anything, even for a good cause.

"Let me write. I will come in the kitchen as soon as I am done," I said, giving Teddy to my mom. I needed no distractions.

"Okay." She took him into the kitchen with her. "Ted, we know when we are not wanted," she said loudly.

"Oh, my gosh, it's not like that at all. I love you both."

The mind of an anorexic—what a dangerous place that is. I typed:

We all feel worthless sometimes, but the level I felt was almost indescribable. It's that feeling of being completely empty. Empty of food as fuel. Empty of friends. Empty of happiness. You become convinced you aren't going anywhere. Your dreams won't come true. There is a record player of voices flowing through your head at all times. Why leave the bed? You are garbage. No one cares about you, loves you. How could they? You aren't pretty enough, smart enough, good enough for anyone, anything. They will be better off without you. Everyone will be. That is how you feel. Is it valid? Is it true? You believe it is, it becomes your bible and you treat yourself accordingly. You are too chicken shit to take your own life, so you punish yourself with starvation. You kill yourself with hunger, a slow drawn-out death. You lose your hair, your vision, you even know you look bad, but you can't stop because dammit YOU JUST CAN'T! WHY DOESN'T ANYONE UNDERSTAND THAT?

You question every morsel of food, every crumb. If you ate, not only would you be worthless, but you would be fat on top of it all. Yes, ON TOP OF IT ALL. #MentalHealthAwarenessMonth #AnorexiaAwareness #RecoveryIsPossible

I pressed Post, and then felt a little sad. Remembering those feelings was tough. I still felt like that sometimes, and it's sad. I must not have realized that my face looked strained, which happens when I am thinking deeply.

"Hey, you, Deep in Thought. I could see on Facebook that you are done. Are you still too cool to hang with us?" my mom asked, peering in from the kitchen.

"Stalker," I shouted back as I shut my computer and stood up. "Well, too cool, always," I added, my sarcasm obvious, "but I will make an exception this time."

Spending time with the people I love always makes me feel better.

CHAPTER 6

Vampires Cry Too

Since my intention had always been to work with my dad, when I nabbed an internship at another transportation company, I was excited to spend the summer before my sophomore year learning as much as I could. After my first day, however, I contracted an unusual strain of pinkeye that, as the doctor put it, "makes people in India go blind."

For two months, I knew how those people in India felt. I was, for all intents and purposes, blind; my eyes were red, watery, crusted over, my vision extremely blurred. If that wasn't bad enough, I was dubbed "Grey Goose Patient of the Year," an honor given to whoever made the eye doctor have a big glass of Grey Goose at the end of the day out of pity for that patient. Because he had to perform several eye surgeries on me during this summer for me to avoid going blind—I was guilty as charged! Trust me, I wanted to pound back those drinks with him...

What shit luck, this would only happen to you, I heard playing in my head like a broken record. All summer I hardly ate, but out of pity for *the blind,* no one mentioned it. It was as if I had turned into a vampire and everyone around me accepted it—I mean, being a vampire was trendy anyway, thanks to The Twilight Saga. What vampire do you know that eats food, anyway? Edward Cullen never binged on sundaes and pizza—how do you think he got his famous six-pack abs? So, it made sense that no one bothered me about my intake, and in terms of having everyone off my back about my size, vampire life wasn't too shabby.

There were many stages to my transition into a full-on blood-sucking vampire: (1) The brightness of the sun would burn my eyes, so I had to stay inside in the dark, and (2) after an entire summer indoors, I was as pale as I'd imagine a vampire to be. (3) My dismal mood made me conclude that I didn't like most humans, and it would be easier sucking their blood than befriending them anyway. (Totally kidding on three, but for all you human readers out there, watch your necks at night—Dani Sherman is still on the loose.)

The only good thing about being quarantined was the ample time to think about my life and review the last year at school. I didn't like being far away from home, and now that I had Blake in my life, I didn't want to miss out on what the relationship could blossom into. I hadn't seen Blake all summer due to the highly contagious nature of my eyes and my vampire fangs, which was hard. I didn't want to be far away from him or my parents. I made the decision to apply to transfer to NYU, but it was too late for this semester.

That last semester I lost what was left of my few remaining Babson friends. I was either at class, the library, the gym, or bingeing and purging on laxatives. If I wasn't purging for a whole weekend and studying, I was visiting my family and Blake. When I transferred to NYU mid-sophomore year, it was as if no one had noticed. I had become a loner at Babson, and it wasn't my newfound vampire ways that made me avoid the daylight and all the people participating in it. It was my eating disorder.

X

I loved Manhattan, and NYU, in the Bohemian Lower East Side, felt like a home away from home. I rented an apartment close to campus, and Blake unofficially lived with me most of the time, even though six months into it, I sensed we were better long-distance.

While we had several issues that were just too big for us to work through, one point of contention was my eating disorder. I tried to hide my secret, and I was able to mask my bellyaches as mere bellyaches, but there were other things I couldn't explain, especially with someone living on top of me in a shoebox-sized Manhattan apartment. When Blake wanted to meet up for lunch like so-called "normal couples" tend to do, I'd conveniently have to study in the library. *Conclusion Blake: Duh, Dani doesn't eat lunch.* Dinner every night was sushi: a tuna roll, and seaweed salad, followed by a handful of pretzels for dessert if I was feeling generous with myself. And that was *every* night, which really limits where you can go for date nights. *Conclusion Blake: Dani eats the same thing every day, that's a little odd. Oh, and she doesn't eat very much.* My self-consciousness invaded the bedroom, where we often wound up fighting instead of having sexy time. *Conclusion Blake: Dani really isn't well.*

Finally, after two years, Blake pulled the plug on a relationship that was long dead. "I wish we were just friends again," he admitted to me one day after a fight.

His wish was my command. I broke up with him right after that. How could I be with someone who wanted to be just friends? And the years we were together felt negated when, two weeks later, Blake found a new girlfriend who he said I, too, "would like if I ever met her." Yeah, I am sure I would just *love* her. (Insert gun emoji to my head. At least back when it wasn't on the emoji extinction list.)

As a result of my heartbreak and the stress I put on myself to "finally get down to a weight where I'd be happy," because nothing else seemed to be working, my insomnia worsened. My therapist and I experimented until we found the right dosage of Xanax to quiet the endless streams of rambling thoughts that kept me staring at the ceiling from my bed. We didn't talk about my eating disorder. In fact, we talked about my anxiety over everything *but* food. The only dose of Xanax that would work was 2 mg, an enormous dose for most people. At bedtime, I would take one and breathe a sigh of relief that soon I would be temporarily relieved from my own mind. I would fall asleep, away from my crazy thoughts about food and life, away from the person who needed to be in control and perfect, away in a drug-induced sleep.

I'd had "crazy" thoughts all of my life. "Two anxiety disorders in particular, obsessive compulsive disorder (OCD) and social phobia, commonly occur with anorexia and bulimia," writes author Carolyn Costin.[1] I had both.

My OCD rituals were very particular. I would count numbers, and multiples of 13 had bad juju. I couldn't shut off the lights at 11:13 p.m., 11:26 p.m., etc. I also couldn't do anything a multiple of 13 times. So, I couldn't end my crunches at 13, 26, 39, or 52. I also had to be the last person to shut off the lights or I was convinced that something bad would happen. Before sleep, in order to guard against remaining ugly and fat, oh and a bad athlete (because being a good athlete made everyone proud), I would compulsively chant, "I wish that I was the best athlete in the world, skinniest and prettiest" until I drifted off. That, plus the constant obsessing about every single morsel of food I put in my mouth and planning my binges and purges, left me with little energy for anything else.

My saving grace became the volunteer work I had signed up to do at a homeless shelter called New York Rescue Mission. I served food, talked, and laughed with the people there. The chef was an endearing man, and it wasn't long before I bonded with him and with all the men who lived there. I felt comfortable with them, as well as comforted by them. It was the one time I felt good in my own skin and happy—a sensation that was foreign to me. To them, I was just Dani, a student. I wasn't Dani, the girl who had to do well in school and had great notes to borrow for exams. I was liked for *my* personality, *my* flaws, *my* heart, and it was very refreshing.

Helping people was the first thing in my life, besides starving and pill-popping (making mama proud with this one!), I felt I really excelled at without much effort. *I, Dani Sherman, am good at making people feel good.* That was one thing in my life I was

---

1   Costin, Carolyn. The Eating Disorder Sourcebook, 3rd ed. (*McGraw-Hill Education, 2007*), page 31.

confident in—my ability to make others smile. I filled any free time I had with volunteering activities: serving at the shelter, working in a children's hospital, visiting an elderly lady weekly, tutoring a homeless man—anything to get that smile and have one moment where I didn't hate myself, where I felt worthy. And that moment made everything hopeful, until it passed...

CHAPTER 7

Natural-Born Starver

I had arranged my life to be so isolated and routinized that even NYU became a bore. Needing a change, I pushed myself to graduate a semester early and put college life behind me. Now I could work with my father, keep volunteering, and focus on things that I believed were *really* important.

Elizabeth had also transferred to NYU and lived close to my apartment. At first, this excited me; I craved the relationship we'd had in high school or at least the idea of it. For years, I hadn't let myself have any kind of new friend or let anyone get too close besides Blake; my eating disorder didn't let me—maybe that was why long-distance was better for us. I missed having a real friend, a confidante.

Elizabeth was a safe friend to have, in that she never said anything about my eating that left me uncomfortable, *ever*. She didn't notice when I gained or lost weight. She didn't notice the way I started binge-drinking in public to avoid eating. Maybe not noticing was not caring, but I didn't mind. In fact, I preferred it. It was a relief that someone remained tight-lipped and nonjudgmental about all my strange behaviors toward eating.

However, our new relationship didn't match what was in my head. Rather than a best friend, I became a mother figure, and, like a daughter, she was annoyed and irritated by my concern. I couldn't help voicing my feelings because my need to protect her, as an empath, trumped caring about her reaction. I was so worried about her. I was always terrified around her, like I had just come into contact with some kind of foreign, multi-headed, fire-breathing dragon that needed to be protected or it would catch itself on fire. What I didn't realize was that, by protecting her, I was getting burned too.

"Lizzie, what are you doing tonight?" I asked one night after work, when I was picking up Teddy. Elizabeth had dog-sat as a favor that day. Her brown hair was in a high bun on top of her head, her blue eyes bloodshot from the weed she'd just smoked.

"I may meet this guy for a date," she said nonchalantly, taking another hit from her bong. A swirl of gray and white smoke filled the room.

"Maybe you shouldn't, you seem a little schwasted," I said, half-joking. I mean, she could handle her weed, but she looked like she was about to pass out, making me think that she'd taken something else before the weed that wasn't agreeing with her. In fact, I could probably snap my fingers in front of her eyes, and I didn't think she would notice...or she would think they were flying birds or something *way* trippy.

I was about to test my theory when she snapped, "I am fine, Dan." Then she rose from her bed and stretched. "You don't even smoke, so you can't judge," she mumbled as Teddy gnawed at one of her shoes in the corner.

"True." I paused, thinking how I feared being judged and didn't want to do that to someone else. "Well, I'm heading back to my apartment now."

"I'll come out with you," she said. "I need to meet my date." Even though she was speaking to me, her eyes drifted in the other direction. I nodded and grabbed Ted and his leash.

We walked out of her apartment, me cradling Teddy, leash wrapped around my arm like a snake. I followed her messy bun to the elevator. She pushed the down button, and we waited in silence. Out of the corner of my eye, I saw her yawn again and rub her high, sleep-ridden eyes.

"Lizzie, I don't mean to be annoying, but are you sure you didn't take something else? You're so sleepy. Why don't you meet this guy another time?"

I hated that she was meeting this random stranger off a dating app while she was so out of it. As my worried mind began to wander to a scenario of me receiving a late-night call about my friend's murder, I felt a sting across my cheek.

"Ouch, what in the actual fuck? Did you just slap me, Lizzie?"

At that moment, the elevator door closed, and like magic, she was gone. I could see the red outline of her hand on my raw cheek in my reflection in the polished metal elevator doors. Shocked and stinging, I still couldn't shake the picture of her being attacked by this "date," so down the stairs I galloped.

When I got to the lobby, I sprinted outside and followed her to a yellow cab. "Lizzie," I begged, grabbing her shoulder in a last-ditch effort to convince her not to go. She turned around and bit me. I winced and drew back my wounded hand, protectively turning my body away from her like a turtle retreating into its shell. When I turned back in her direction, I saw the cab pull away, fumes trailing in gray and white, like Elizabeth's hazy bong smoke.

"Did that just happen?" I asked Teddy. What was I supposed to do now? I knew the answer: go home and starve my emotions away.

A month later, I relocated to New York's Upper East Side, moving closer to work and giving me some much-needed space away from Elizabeth, but our paths would cross again—because they always did seem to reticulate. This time, a shared car service to a mutual family friend's daughter's bat mitzvah did our bidding.

We arrived at cocktail hour, greeting our families and friends with hugs and kisses, me putting on my best fake "everything is great" pageant smile. And I made sure my "Little Miss Starver" pageant ribbon was not around my torso. It was the usual plan—avoid food and just drink, or have one in my hand to avoid the question about what was being put into my mouth.

I put some appetizers on a plate and arranged them strategically as if I had eaten some of them.

I had lost more weight since college graduation. Since I'd started working, I had kept extra thin by never eating during the day and overloading myself with work and volunteering as distractions. Since by nature I am usually so worried about everyone else that I often conveniently forget about myself, this dieting strategy was really easy. In addition to being a naturally good people helper, I was a natural-born starver.

I finished my first drink and headed into the main ballroom, where the music was blasting Corona's "This Is the Rhythm of the Night" and seventh-graders were rushing the dance floor. I saw Elizabeth in my periphery; her hands were in the air and she was following the crowd. I turned around, following her with my eyes. Elizabeth was acting bizarre, and not in an *I-am-judging-you-because-you-are-weird* way, but in a *WTF-is-she-on-I-am-afraid-for-her-safety-and-the-safety-of-others* way. She was so into the music that she made a beeline to the stage, hopped on, and was dancing with the thirteen-year-olds. A Hawaiian lei encircled her neck and big yellow sunglasses were propped on her nose. Each thrust and gyration of her hips made me nervous in a no-not-again way. A thirteen-year-old boy with thick black glasses was standing beside her, and she grabbed his hands and started twirling him in circles. His night was made. I laughed but felt this weird fear. Glancing at the scar of her bite mark on my hand, I placed my other hand over it—as if hiding it would make the memory and bad feelings go away.

"Lizzie sure is having fun," I whispered to my mom, trying to see if she noticed anything odd too. Maybe I was just looking for it?

My mom turned her head toward the stage, where Elizabeth was now sloppily doing the Macarena. She put her right arm, facing down, in front of her, matching her left arm. Then her hands went to her hips, and she shook her butt wildly. My mom cringed as Elizabeth's low-cut dress exposed the cup of her black bra.

"Oh boy," my mom said, walking up to Lizzy's mom. Words were exchanged between the two.

Not long after, and conveniently (for me) just before the main course was served, Elizabeth's parents declared that it was okay for us to leave without being rude. Like hint, hint—leave now! They weren't wrong, either. We were probably being ruder by staying; between my nervous energy and Elizabeth's odd behavior, it was clearly time for us to go. Luckily for Elizabeth's parents, I'd take chaperoning hot-mess-express Elizabeth over awkwardly picking around food with a table of people watching me any day.

On the way home, I tried making small talk with Elizabeth, "So this was a fun night. Did you get any of those thirteen-year-olds' numbers?" I joked, smiling.

"That's not funny," she slurred, the words sounding almost inaudible. Then, suddenly, she began vomiting all over herself in the backseat of the town car. I cleaned her up the best I could, let her pass out on my lap, and stroked her beautiful brown hair, which smelled strongly of vomit and hard alcohol. In that moment, it was obvious that her spiral was as deep as mine.

"Stay strong, Lizzie," I said, kissing her on the forehead. "You are going to be okay."

Oh, how I wished someone would tell me the same.

FULL LIFE, AUGUST 2013

My feet touched the soft sand, searching for shells between my toes. My brown curls spiraled wildly in the wind. The sun hit my face, accentuating the freckles on my cheeks. The freckles would soon blend together, forming a sun-kissed tan. This hadn't happened in a while.

"This feels nice," I said, as I continued walking on the sandy beach. The waves hit, a rhythmic up and down, thrashing on the shore.

"Yes, this is called the ocean. This is called the sand. That is the sun. *Relaxation*...what a concept," my boyfriend, Sebastian, quipped, pointing to each as he made fun of my work-obsessed type-A mentality.

"*Really?* I will have to add those words to my vocabulary. What was the first one, *ocean?*" I quipped back, giving a sarcastic smile as we kept walking toward my parents, who were working at our barbecue setup on the beach.

"Nantucket is really beautiful, isn't it?" I said, looking at Sebastian's deep brown eyes. "I have a memory from when I was a little girl of my grandpa finding my cousins and me purple sand. I thought it was the coolest thing I ever saw. No one remembers it except me and one cousin, but we are so sure it happened."

"Knowing your grandpa, he probably dyed the sand purple and told you girls it was like that," my dad said, putting a grilled hot dog on a bun and squirting ketchup on it.

"No, I remember digging to get to it. It happened." I placed a turkey burger with American cheese on a bun, sat on my towel, and bit into the juicy summer favorite. I adjusted my blue-and-white-striped bikini, giving myself props for the festive attempt on this Fourth of July. "I never thought I would get to this place—eating a burger in a bikini. Scandalous," I said, resting my head on Sebastian's shoulder, an invitation for a kiss.

"You got to learn to be a little easier on yourself, kid," my mom said, throwing a fry and hitting me in the chest. (No cereal available.)

"Well, you know what they say, practice makes perfect, and I am practicing right now." I threw a fry back at her. "Boom, right in the head."

Later that day, I decided to write a post, accompanied by a picture of a little kid in Batman garb with the quote: "The most important thing in life is to be yourself. Unless you can be Batman. Always be Batman."

"The problem is these kids are smart, but their emotional temperament can't and shouldn't have to handle this kind of responsibility or pressure. Their eating disorder behaviors are often the signals telling others 'Help me! I can't handle all of this, and I can't tell you that.' "
—Carolyn Costin, *The Eating Disorder Sourcebook*

There is just so much that one person can do. It's easy to put a lot of pressure on yourself and very hard to ask for help—especially as someone who doesn't like to bother anyone and feels responsible for every single situation put in front of her. I personally didn't ask for help for so long because I felt like I would be a burden to my family and an utter disappointment. My control of food was my outlet as everything else seemed so out of control, and eventually I became isolated in my own ED world in order to hold onto some kind of false power. If something is too much, tell someone. It's not a disappointment and it's totally okay to not be able to take on the world all of the time—we are not bionic and have no superhero powers like Batman (unfortunately because that would be kind of awesome ;)). Be you! That is acting like a true superhero! My superhero power is my empathy; what is yours?

Fireworks were starting to go off. "So beautiful," I said under my breath. I went outside to watch them with my parents and Sebastian. What a difference a year makes.

CHAPTER 8

The Answer, Alex Trebek, Is What Is Total Destruction?

With Blake in the rearview mirror, any speck of a social life now buried, and an equally troubled best friend, all I had to lean on was Teddy, volunteering, and work—the latter being my main priority. My master plan had come to fruition: my father hired me immediately after graduation from NYU. It didn't occur to me how against the idea he was until he treated me like crap. Today he admits that, during those first three months, he was a complete asshole—his words, not mine (at least to his face)—in the hope that he would break me down and I would be miserable enough to change my mind. Clearly, he didn't know how strong-willed I was. He wasn't privy to how much pain, torture, self-control, discipline, and pure will one must have to starve oneself. This isn't to say his strictness didn't take its toll on me.

"Dani, this isn't how I told you to do this," my dad said, brows furrowed, looking over how I'd closed out the day before.

"Yes, but it's easier for me to use my scientific calculator then an adding machine. I just figured the Excel spreadsheet that I created would be a new way to double-check too, bringing you into the twenty-first century. You just need to plug numbers in and the formula does the work for you." I paused, looking up at him, getting nervous. "I was just trying something new, if that's alright, of course." I finished, taking a deep breath in, sensing maybe it wasn't "alright." This was not the reaction I was expecting.

"No, it's not, Dani. Do it again. I need adding tape, that's how I do things."

"Alright, I will do it again. Sorry."

"If you are not going to listen, don't work for me. Bottom line."

"I know, I know, I get it. I am sorry, I am doing it again right now," I said, soothingly.

My dad was my very first boss, but at a certain point, it became hard for me to separate the two relationships. So, instead of trying to put myself in my father's shoes—appreciating his need to keep up a tough profile to employees, avoid rumors of nepotism or favoritism, and train me to act like an employee—I believed his behavior toward me was an indication that he thought I was inept, unlovable, an embarrassment, and a total fuck-up.

ED was, of course, egging these thoughts on: *You will never be as good as he wants you to be. He doesn't love you. You do everything wrong. You're a disappointment to him.*

I doubled down on my work and increased my hours, trying to show myself and everyone else that I wasn't a spoiled girl doing nothing while she collects Daddy's paychecks. I would earn my keep in sweat and time and be the best worker anyone in the company had ever seen. What I didn't know was that my father's plan was the same as mine, in the beginning. He was attempting to beat any hint of entitlement out of me by treating me like absolute shit for the first couple of months. Call it a biological probation period. But I wasn't the personality type that needed that push. I didn't have any entitlement to begin with! To make matters worse, my dad lashes out when he can't control things, while I lash inward at myself. I probably inherited this need to control from him, but ultimately him yelling at me only increased my self-hate. Between his high expectations and my self-beatings, I worked twelve- to fourteen-hour days, losing not only additional pounds, but also any semblance of a balanced life.

After the first year, my father seemed to accept me and even started to depend on me, but I still felt like I had so much to prove. My objective became to say yes to everything.

"Dani, can you finish these bank statements by the end of the night?"

"Yes."

"Dani, can you stay late and show the dispatchers how to use the new cashiering app?"

"Yes."

"Dani, can you do a headstand on your desk and touch your nose?"

"Of course I can. And I can do a cartwheel to top it off." I would say yes to everything, even if it seemed impossible, and would get it done with that A-plus cherry on top I was so used to adding.

I woke up every morning at five, brushed my teeth, and threw my hair into a messy bun. I hailed a cab, getting to work by six at the latest, and worked until at least six-thirty at night with no breaks. I didn't eat breakfast or lunch. My dad and I shared an office, and he observed that I never ate, but he stopped saying anything after a while. Sometimes I would order a sandwich and throw it out, so he would think I was eating. And if he had ever ventured to comment, I would have cut him off, threatened to leave, or snapped, completely freaking the fuck out, defending my anorexia like my unborn child. It was my everything.

To further prove myself, I went into the office on weekends and never took a vacation. I didn't think I deserved one. This pattern went on for four long, unhealthy years. I had been sick for most of my life, but this period was rock bottom. I was a full-fledged adult with real responsibilities. Living independently with my own money made it so much easier to hide my disorder. I could keep certain odd and dangerous behaviors as private as I wanted to. I was also old enough now to accompany my ED with some fun new addictions—but I'm getting ahead of myself.

During this time, I started exploring new weight-loss techniques, starting with an over-the-phone weight-loss center that sent prepackaged foods. This was something I wouldn't have been able to do as a younger person without the consent of my parents. But with no supervision, I was free to follow the 1,200-calorie menu, making sure I didn't mix up meals, doing whatever I wanted with them—eat them or throw them in the trash unopened. I lied to my meal counselor about my starting weight and how much I would lose each week—easy-peasy over the phone.

This diet was an OCD dream. I put everything in the kitchen in the order of the days of the week and looked up all the foods online during the day and thought about them constantly, checking back with the menu just in case I had made a mistake and mixed up days, meals, etc. I couldn't afford an extra calorie. This was the first time I allowed myself to eat semi-normal foods in minuscule portions— pasta, pizza, and hamburgers—although I abstained from all the snacks and vegetables they recommended to keep you feeling full and able to stick to the diet. I didn't need that full feeling—in fact, I craved the empty. In addition, I had an elliptical in my apartment and would often use it for up to ninety minutes in the morning or when I came home from work at night to compensate for what I was eating.

I could tell by how my clothing fit that I had lost a few pounds, but predictably, after two months, I found myself eating the entire two weeks' planned meals in one sitting. Done in by a fridge filled to the brim with frozen blueberry pancakes and veggie sausage, breakfast sandwiches, the beef and cheese sliders, beef chow mein. The boxes of yummy food just kept going—food I hadn't eaten since I was a child, food I had recently tried again, none of which, to my disappointment, I disliked. My fridge wasn't used to being that full, and the sight made me salivate like a rabid animal.

One night, I came home from work, my stomach growling like Teddy at a bigger dog, trying to prove itself more powerful than my will. *It was.*

"Oy, Ted, I think I am just going to eat right now," I said, looking down at him as if to get his approval. He looked back like he always did—his little black beady eyes staring, hoping I'd continue petting him.

"I'll cuddle in a second. Right now, it's time for Mommy to eat."

I swung the fridge open. "It seems tonight we have chicken fettuccine; how very Italiano of us. Right, Ted?" I double-checked the menu posted on the fridge to make sure fettuccine was what I was supposed to have—even though I had checked the menu about four billion times (only exaggerating by a billion or two) that day.

In the background, Alex Trebek pronounced, "On September 1, 1715, Louis the Fourteenth died in this city, site of a fabulous palace he built."

I put the meal in the microwave. As it heated, I readied the salt and silverware. Then *beep, beep, beep*—done. "What is Versailles?" answered a contestant. I grabbed one noodle and slurped it up, the rich, creamy, buttery sauce hitting my tongue.

"Wow, Ted, this is delicious," I said as I took the plate to the couch. I tried to eat slowly and savor each bite, twirling the noodles with my tongue and sucking each one. I was *so* hungry, and the taste was so good that I couldn't control myself. To savor each noodle one by one was an impossible feat. Before I knew it, the plate was empty, but unfortunately, I wasn't full. I looked at the clock shining brightly in front of me. Not even eight o'clock! How would I wait out the whole night before I could eat again?

I looked at the TV in front of me and scowled at the plastic image of Alex Trebek. "Sakura cheese from Hokkaido is a soft cheese flavored with leaves from this fruit tree. Yes, Maria."

"What is cherry?" the woman answered confidently, earning six hundred dollars.

Despite my effort to focus on the TV, all I could think about was the food in the fridge, all that delicious food calling to me. I tapped my fingers against the couch. I looked down to find Ted fighting to get up onto the couch, begging with his little paws. Whose struggle was greater right now, his or mine? *Mine.*

Ignoring his pleas, I beelined to the fridge, selected a macaroni and cheese, and proceeded to shovel it into my mouth, barely out of the microwave. I was eating so fast I hardly tasted it.

Then more—Salisbury steak and cheese enchiladas—straight from the microwave to my mouth. I couldn't even taste the flavors, and I burned the roof of my mouth on the cheese enchiladas because I didn't let them cool down. Then to the pantry, one bag of cheese curls, followed by bruschetta veggie chips, a pumpkin loaf, two cinnamon rolls… I couldn't help it. By the time I came out of my food trance, it was a half-hour later, my mouth was on fire, and almost all the food in the fridge was gone. I covered my mouth with my shaky hands. They were sticky from the cruddy cinnamon buns, and I felt so nauseated, my stomach ballooned. I needed to pop it—deflate it back to its normal size.

In a fit of anger, I grabbed the small amount of food that was left, threw it into a garbage bag, and shoved it down the incinerator chute in the hall.

"What did I do, Ted?" I said, holding my bloated stomach and swaying back and forth to try to ease the pain. There was only one solution. I climbed to the top of my closet and opened my Louis Vuitton tote, where I kept my stash. Ninety Dulcolax laxative pills! One by one, I popped them. I gagged a few times, but I succeeded; I always did. I lay down nauseated, head pounding, and closed my eyes. I drifted off into a horrible sweaty sleep. Sweat soaked through my pajamas and onto my mattress, staining it. Hours later when I woke, it was the middle of the night, and I lurched to the bathroom, throwing up with bursts of terrible diarrhea, sometimes at the same time.

Sitting on the toilet with a garbage pail filled to the brim with vomit at 1:09 a.m., I muttered to myself: "Clue: This girl screwed up bingeing on a whole two weeks' worth of meals. She is a complete loser and failure." I paused looking around as if waiting for a *Jeopardy* contestant to appear by the toilet. "Yes, Dani," I mocked Alex Trebek. "The answer, Alex, is Who Is Danielle Sherman?" I laughed crazily as tears filled my eyes.

In the morning, my whole body ached, and my eyes were bloodshot; bags beneath them drooped to my cheekbones. But my stomach was no longer enlarged. It was worth it.

I did this twice in a week, until I cancelled my phone-in diet membership due to my lack of self-control. This wasn't going to work. It was too tempting to binge with all of that food sitting in the fridge, taunting me with its tastes, textures, presentation. The solution was to buy *just one* diet microwaveable meal a day; that was all the food that would be allowed in my apartment and for me to eat. Bingeing would be a last resort—almost impossible to do on a whim. So that's what I did.

Often, I would come home shaken from something that had happened at work. Most of the time, my angst was about a disagreement with my dad over something so simple as a miscalculation or a typo. He would point out the transgression so I "wouldn't do it again," but I would belittle myself for making those mistakes and being incompetent.

The stress of the day, combined with the fear of being unable to sleep on an empty stomach, drove me to the bottle. Once home, I would ceremoniously take out a bottle of wine and pour myself a glass, but that alone did not suffice. Wine was easy. For a natural-born starver, hunger was pretty easy. I needed something to make me *really* feel pain. So I turned to another type of self-destruction, cutting.

The first time I placed a knife against my lower back above my butt and laid down on it, I was nervous, but excited, like going down a roller coaster for the first time. I was feeling hopeless, stuck in my eating habits, miserable. So many emotions, yet nothing at all. The knife in my skin was punishment, yet also a release. With the blood that dripped out of my back, so did a little bit of my inner turmoil. The pain felt so good, so relieving. *I deserved it.*

After cutting, I'd grab my Xanax and wash it down with wine to the point of delirium, heat up the one diet microwavable meal I'd bought that day, and pick at it as I passed out. Sometimes I'd wake up to discover I'd somehow gotten myself into bed. Other times, I'd still be on the couch, my face pressed into the cushion where I usually cuddled with Teddy. Wherever I was, somehow Teddy would find me and lie with me or guard the room I slept in, as if he sensed that something bad was happening.

This combination proved treacherous. One morning, I woke up with a burn on my face the size of a pancake.

"I got hit with a hot ladle at the shelter," I explained to my parents.

"That's only something that would happen to you," my dad said, as he took a sip of his Coors Light beer, knowing I could run on the klutzy side at times.

I'd met my parents at a Greek restaurant down the street from where I lived—just to say hi; I'd told them I'd already eaten.

"That looks really bad. I think we should put Aquaphor on it, and, Dan, you really have to be more careful," my mom said, sizing up the burn.

"Well, you know the movie *The Hangover* is very popular, so in the spirit of it, I thought I should really embody Mike Tyson—you know, the face tattoo," I quipped as I played with the salt and pepper shakers, smiling at my witty joke.

"Not funny, Dan," my mom retorted, rolling her eyes as she put a forkful of Greek salad into her mouth.

✕

How did I really get that burn?

"I am like pure badass right now, Ted. You have a badass mom, like so badass. I can party with Lil Wayne and his 'purple drank[2]' level."

That's what I remember saying to Ted as I'd headed to the kitchen to heat up my meal the day before.

The shepherd's pie box instructions said to heat the pie in the microwave for two minutes and open the microwave door as the timer went off. I danced around in a circle, left hand waving in the air, right hand wrapped around the foil of a bottle of Rosé, as I waited for the microwave to heat up my dinner. I took one last swig before opening the microwave. I vaguely remember hearing the timer go off, me opening the door nonchalantly, and the scalding pie filling exploding in my face. I was so drunk and high on Xanax that it seemed comical. I laughed, feeling the hot pie mash on my skin. Then, as it blinded me, I tripped over my own feet while attempting to take another swig of wine straight from the bottle.

Then everything went black.

The next morning, I woke up on the kitchen floor in a puddle of wine. Not a good look. I felt horrible, hung-over, and then there was this terrible burning sensation on my face. I took my right hand and grabbed my eye—that didn't help. I pulled myself up and went to my bedroom. That is when I took one glance in the mirror and saw a raw hot-pink ring around my eye.

This is just what I need, something to make me look uglier and draw more attention to my face. Something to let the world really know how messed-up I am. My skinny body is not enough.

✕

Telling my parents that I was accidentally hit with a hot ladle at a shelter was not too far-fetched. I did have accidents at the shelters I served at—my frail, easy-to-bruise body bumping into pots, pans, and tables, all the time. I would get comments from residents at the shelter, telling me to stop dishing them food because I could use it for myself.

---

2 According to Wikipedia, purple drank is a recreational drug which includes a prescription-strength cough syrup mixed with a carbonated soft drink. The mixture became popular in the hip hop community in the southern United States in the 1990s.

I even once had an old lady say, "I could tell you're Jewish because you look like you were in a concentration camp."

"Oh," was all I could muster in response, a little, and probably understandably, taken aback.

As messed-up as that was to say, and politically incorrect at that, I mean this elder woman suffered from dementia and God knows what else, but the one thing she got right was that I was scary skinny.

On several occasions, I passed out. The steaming heat of the food I was serving, combined with how weak I was from not eating or hydrating myself adequately, did me in. Here I was, an adult, twenty-five years old, and I couldn't even volunteer without assistance anymore. I was falling apart.

I have become a burden. People who need help are starting to want to help me. I am a failure, and I should just disappear. The lead volunteer of the group threatened to call an ambulance after I almost passed out on the line and had to lie down on the shelter floor to avoid free-falling. Volunteers and shelter residents alike surrounded me, eyes wide and concerned—me, guiltily taking the last paper cup we had in supply because I needed the water for myself. A thirsty little boy had to drink from his cupped hands because I couldn't feed myself properly. I never hated myself more than I did in that moment.

After that, I was told that if I fainted again it would be reported to the volunteer organization and be put on my records (whatever that meant, it freaked me out enough to heed the warning). So, on two separate occasions after that, I left the serving line, complaining of a made-up stomachache, and hid in the bathroom, where I lay on the filthy floor, waiting for the light-headed feeling to pass and praying that a roach wouldn't attack me, all to avoid being "reported." It got to the point where I had to give up volunteering or I was sure to be discovered—caught red-handed, outed as an anorexic.

Around the same time, Mom began begging me to make an appointment with our family doctor.

It had been two years since I'd gone to a doctor. My body was so frail, I couldn't hide my illness from a professional anymore. I knew because I had already tried that. The scale was sure to give me away, just like last time...

Dr. Lev was my parents' physician. My father, figuring he was due for a physical, said we should go together before work. This idea had my mom's name written all over it, but I agreed to get both of them off my back.

While my father read a magazine in the waiting room, I was in a gown being forced onto a scale. Ninety-three pounds, which for my age, twenty-three, and build was way too light. The doctor asked about my stress level and berated me for taking Xanax for my anxiety.

"Kids are so hard on themselves these days. I don't know why you guys put so much pressure on yourselves." His patronizing, all-knowing tone reminded me of why I hated doctors. I sat there silently, watching his mouth move but muting the sounds. *How could he not understand that I couldn't fall asleep? I would be up thinking about everything, and without something to take the edge off, I would be up all night.* This was my worst fear.

I was petrified of not being able to sleep. The idea that I would be held hostage to my thoughts all night, unable to press my brain's shutdown button, preoccupied my day. I might as well have been tied down to my bed and forced to watch heinous images roll like an old-fashioned film reel. Sleep was obviously one of the best ways to not eat, to make the dreaded hours pass, to escape. So I would swallow 2 mg of Xanax, many times 3 mg (abusing it), just to be sure I would conk out into a dreamless state, oblivious to whatever my unconscious mind wanted to scream at me. And I wasn't opposed to dangerously chasing the pill with white wine. In fact, it was my chaser every night, without fail.

If I didn't take my Xanax-wine cocktail and couldn't sleep, I would work out on the elliptical trainer for ninety minutes, usually starting at midnight. Feet not leaving the pedals, my legs went up and down in one fluid movement. I could hear the machine squeaking, then I'd reverse and pedal backward, calves and quads burning. I'd watch television shows I'd recorded to distract myself. I would get off, examine my bulge, and then hop back on in disgust and work out for another hour and a half. I'd frustratedly watch the clock move from three five, at which time I'd head into the shower and then off to work.

Dr. Lev brought me back from my deep thoughts to his examining room as I heard him ask, "Can I tell your father about your low weight?" I hesitated, replaying the words in my mind slower, "Tell my father about my low weight." *Hell, to the no! Who did this guy think he was?*

I managed to stutter, "No, but thanks, I will make everything better." *It was my private business. Was he going to tell?*

For the next twenty minutes, I waited outside the door while the doctor examined my dad, anxious that he would reveal my secret. Lucky for me, he didn't. This is another aspect of having an eating disorder in adulthood. There is no medical disclosure to parents.

So, as any crafty anorexic would do, I didn't go to a doctor for two years, especially since I assumed I was at a dangerously low weight now, much lower than when I was twenty-three. No way would I risk being forced into a hospital for a seventy-two-hour hold. I saw what they did to Britney Spears. Thanks, but no thanks! To appease my worried mother, I lied. "I went to the doctor," I explained. "He said I was anemic, which is why I'm sometimes weak and tired and bruise so easily."

As my lying escalated, my health diminished. And I *really* didn't think I could change anything, nor was I sure I wanted to...

FULL LIFE, AUGUST 2013

Where does ED come from? What made him find me, out of everyone in third grade? I was so young, no curves yet, my diet and weight loss didn't have to do with "feeling fat" at the time. Yet I was restricting food the only way I knew how, limiting my peanut butter and jelly sandwiches and avoiding what I believed to be fattening foods like French fries. I decided to ask my mom about it.

It was a warm August afternoon. The sun shone strong, heat hitting me hard with each step I took to meet my mom at Green Kitchen, a diner on the Upper East Side. I gave her a sweaty hug, and we browsed the menu, taking sips of water.

"I will have an egg-white wrap with turkey and American cheese with a side salad, please," I said to the waiter as he jotted down my request on a notepad.

"I will have a chicken salad wrap, please," my mom chimed in.

"Fries or side salad?" the waiter asked.

"Fries," my mom answered and handed the waiter our menus.

"I love Saturdays," I said. "I got to sleep in this morning, and it was pretty glorious."

"I bet."

"Mom, I have a question for you," I said, taking my hair in my hands. "So I have been doing some reading, and I am pretty sure Bummy [the nickname for my great-grandmother] had an eating disorder."

Mounting evidence shows that genetics play a part in eating disorders. It is not at all uncommon for eating disorders to run in families. It skipped my mom, but I remember my great-grandma talking about food all the time. She would comment about her weight and how thin or fat everyone was, how little she weighed, and last, how her sister was a food pusher.

When I visited her in the nursing home as she got older, she would ask me to put on lipstick, handing me a tacky bright pink hue so she could "show me off." How I was as a person was never emphasized. What was important to her was what I physically looked like. That form of acceptance made me feel bad about myself and uncomfortable.

That's just what she valued above anything else; however, people with anorexia vary on their values, like all human beings do. Just because we are obsessed with being skinny, that doesn't mean it is the most important thing to us in other people. I, for one, care so much more about people's insides than their physiques—when judging people, I don't look twice at their appearance. But for my great-grandmother, being beautiful and thin was everything.

"Mom, do you think anyone else in our family has a problem like that?"

To my surprise, she answered, "Well, there was *my* mom."

My grandmother had died of cancer when I was just two years old, so unfortunately, I didn't know her very well. My mom told me that she suffered "the other way" with binge-eating disorder. My mom said that, although she would never see her eating, my grandmother gained a lot of weight and became very heavy over the years. Her choice phrase for this behavior was "closet eating."

Our orders came to the table, placed with a thump in front of us. I poured honey mustard dressing on my side salad and ate a forkful. "I'm hungry," I said taking another bite.

"Me too!" my mom agreed.

Later that day, I posted on my Living a FULL Life Facebook page:

> *"Eating disorders are like a gun that's formed by genetics, loaded by a culture and family ideals, and triggered by unbearable distress."*
> —Aimee Liu

> *Today load your gun with* FULLets *(my word for encouraging bullets) and shoot toward loving yourself. Think of one characteristic that makes you feel special and hone in on that quality. Then take that thought and trigger a beautiFULL day.*

I clicked Post and sat back on the couch, where Teddy curled next to me in a little ball, face pressing against my side.

"Let's watch a movie, Ted," I said, picking him up and placing him on top of me, sinking both of us deeper into the cushions of the couch, getting comfortable. "We are allowed to rest sometimes. We deserve it."

The summer I was twenty-four, persuaded by their constant urging (borderline nagging), I finally agreed to visit my parents and spend the night out in Sag Harbor where they rented a house for the summer. By the time I got there, after working all morning, it was Saturday night, just in time for dinner. *Oh joy,* I bet you could imagine my *complete* thrill. My parents had assured me we were going to have a healthy meal, knowing I wouldn't eat anything fatty or "unsafe."

To honor their promise, Mom prepared steamed sole, jasmine rice, and steamed mixed vegetables. When I started eating, something almost magical happened. That little voice taunting me quieted down. It was as if someone turned the volume down a couple of notches for once. I drank wine and actually let myself *eat* instead of *pick*. With my mom's urging, I even tasted the rice, then let myself have all of it, slowly, hands shaking from anxiety—but I did it.

That night, I ate every last bit on my plate and laughed for the first time in a long while. I even let myself have a small slice of pound cake for dessert. As the soft, sweet taste hit my taste buds, I smiled. I could see in their eyes how happy my parents were that I was eating. The normal tense vibe that surrounded mealtime with them was lifted, and we were actually enjoying each other's company.

After dessert, I went to my room and curled up on my side, trying to fall asleep before the guilt over what I'd just consumed sank in. But I couldn't shut my brain off, and my head started spinning with neurotic thoughts. I didn't want to go home tomorrow. I didn't want to go back into isolation. I didn't want be alone with myself anymore. That's where the damage is done and the eating disorder breeds itself. I couldn't be trusted alone. I couldn't help but hurt myself. I didn't want to go back to the way things were, just a couple of hours, minutes, seconds before dinner.

But why did I have to feel so guilty about everything I'd just consumed? I couldn't help but think about the ways I was going to burn off all the calories. *Do rounds of twenty crunches.* I gently pulled my abdominals inward, curled up and forward so that my head, neck, and shoulder blades lifted off the floor. Held for a moment at the top of the movement and then lowered slowly back down. *Repeated, times twenty.* Out of breath.

I couldn't escape my thoughts. *Would I ever be able to?* Another round of twenty crunches. Toss and turn, toss turn, toss turn. After a few hours, I'd had enough; I went to my parents' room, quietly opening the door, and tapped my sleeping mom's shoulder.

"Can I come into your bed? I can't sleep," I whispered, like a five-year-old afraid of monsters in the closet. And I *was* afraid of a monster; I was afraid of anorexia. I just wasn't aware of it yet, which made me afraid of myself.

"Sure," my mom said, then added, after a pause, "Are you okay?" She knew the answer; her daughter hadn't been okay in years.

"I don't know, Mom," I said, snuggling into her arms. As I closed my eyes to try to finally sleep, I felt a wet spot on my cheek. Tears. Like a little girl, I slept there all night cuddled in my mom's arms.

The next day was Sunday. Time for me to go back to the city—back to reality. I was planning to get back early enough to put in some Sunday hours at the office. Really, I'd arranged this to avoid eating breakfast or lunch with my parents, but a feeling of sadness made my skin crawl. I needed to go, stay—I debated back and forth between the two. Go, get my work done, then use the elliptical, and burn the extra calories I'd consumed last night. Plus, I wouldn't have to eat anything today. Or stay. I couldn't think of any calorie-saving benefits, except something was telling me to *just stay* and pulling me a little more toward that.

"Can I go home later today?" I asked my parents. They, of course, said yes. They were incredibly happy that I would be spending the day with them, since I was such a loner these days.

Since I had the courage to do that, maybe I had it in me to do *this*.

"Mom, I have something, I think, never mind," I said, fiddling with my fingers behind my back.

"What, Dan?" My mom's voice sounded desperate to pull any morsel of information out of me. Seeing her sick child and not knowing what to do killed her, and I could tell. I felt terrible about it. That's why I generally stayed away—that, *and* to avoid eating or hearing any unwanted comments about my weight.

"I need to show you something. Come upstairs," I said, motioning for her to follow me up the spiral stairs of my parents' house. Suddenly my body seemed to be moving in slow motion.

There was no gravity and each step, each stair, each little movement felt as if I were floating. What was I about to do?

In my childhood bedroom, I plopped down flat on my belly, and pulled down my pants, eyes closed to avoid Mom's initial reaction. I showed her the cuts that lined my butt from my nightly cutting ritual. I showed her the scars, like permanent tattoos of self-hate, on my back.

At first, she didn't say anything, and just traced the scars with her hands as if mystified. Shocked. It seemed like an eternity before she spoke. "Dani, you can't do this to yourself anymore." She paused, trying to think of what else she should say. What was the appropriate thing to say in this type of situation? She had no idea. Neither did I; nothing was going to make this better. "You can't keep hurting yourself," she repeated, still examining the cuts.

"I'm sorry. I know I have to stop."

"Dan, I think you need more help. Maybe we need to up your sessions with Dr. Blatter, or maybe you should try going on medication. I don't know why you won't give it a shot. They don't turn you into a robot and..."

"I promise. I am going to handle it," I replied meekly, interrupting her before she could give more suggestions. All I could think after my confession was, *how will I survive without my coping mechanisms?* And I really wanted to stop these behaviors at times like these, but at other times, I wanted to keep doing them. I wanted to keep disappearing until I vanished completely. I thought about dying a lot. I would never admit this to her, but there was something comforting, relieving about ending it all. Putting a permanent end to that voice in my head.

My mom looked frightened. I was scared by her reaction, along with the fact that, in that instant, I knew I wasn't ready to give up cutting or my eating disorder. Everything in my head was screaming *NOOOOO, stop talking.*

Throughout that day, my mom and dad rooted me on like my own personal cheerleading squad. I got through a turkey wrap with honey mustard for lunch. It had been several years since I had eaten lunch. When I complained after a couple of bites, feeling full from breakfast—some fruit and cottage cheese—my mom went into rah-rah mode.

"You are so strong. You got this. Just take a couple more bites."

"Yes, I am strong, I can beat this," I said, biting into the wrap one more time.

"You are going to be okay, and I never have been prouder of you!" My mom beamed. She just needed pom-poms.

I found her choice of words ironic—*Strong? Really? I am weak as shit.*

"Thanks," I said as I hesitantly took another bite of the wrap.

When I got back to my apartment later that evening, I felt better about everything. Maybe even hopeful. Maybe cheering helped. I ordered steamed vegetable dumplings and brown rice for dinner, and I went to sleep without abusing alcohol or Xanax outside my normal dosage. I didn't go near my knife. Maybe I was strong. Maybe I could beat this. I could hear my support squad:

Rah-rah strong.

Rah-rah let's go Dani.

Rah-rah you can beat this.

But the next day, when night fell again, after a full day of real-life stress, I was back to dysfunctional Dani. The way I ran my life was the only way I knew, and there was no way I could change. Too uncomfortable, too scary. There was no point in burdening my parents with this issue ever again, because the hurt was so deep it would never go away. Like the sharp knife I used to cut through the skin on my back each night, it was time to cut my parents, the only people left, out of my personal life for good.

Rah-rah goodbye.

CHAPTER 9

The Final Dingle Dangle

I starved myself Saturday through Thursday, so that means I ate *nada, zero, zip, zilch* all day except for one diet microwaveable meal at night. Friday was binge day, so I ate nothing until I got off work. While it felt like the rest of the world was at happy hour, chugging beer, wine, and vodka, I was at home for my private version of the ritual—preparing to *chug* food, swallowing 150 Dulcolax—the primer for my impending binge. The number had increased from 90 to 150 because my body had grown resistant, and now I needed more to have the same effect. (To get an idea of the scope of my addiction, in 2011 alone, I ordered forty-two boxes of 150-count Dulcolax and sixty 48-count boxes of chocolate stimulant ex-lax online.)

A version of this Friday night routine was my very own happy hour. I ordered a cinnamon raisin bagel with peanut butter and jelly, a turkey and cheese bagel, and a fat-free muffin to top it off from the deli downstairs. I sat surrounded by the spread to make it easier to access it during the binge. I'd added my reliable spray butter, pretzels, fat-free cheese, and cereal to the mix.

I started slowly, eating the turkey and cheese on a bagel because that was the less fattening of the two bagel sandwiches and maybe it would fill me up. If it did, I didn't do *that* much damage...at least yet. *Yeah right! Not in binge mode.*

The way I stuffed food in my mouth was animalistic. I was *so* hungry, and it happened *so* fast that I tasted nothing after the first bagel. Then, not too long after—nausea, I felt like I was going to throw up, gosh I wished I could—it would be easier than swallowing all of those pills to get the same result. It hit so hard I fell to the floor in pain. My stomach protruded, and I stayed horizontal, trying to alleviate some of the discomfort. After heavily breathing myself into a light sleep, I awoke to the taste of vomit. I threw up into a trash can (sometimes the diarrhea would start at the same time as the throwing up). The lack of oxygen, gagging, and straining caused my eyes to become bloodshot and my body to convulse, until all that was left was dry-heaving.

This is how I spent the beginning of the weekend, which is why I planned my binges and purges for Friday evenings. Afterward, I would throw any leftover remnants from the binge into a garbage bag, which I'd toss down the garbage chute of my apartment building. All evidence, all proof that it happened, gone. All tempting food in my apartment, gone as well.

For the rest of the weekend, I would catch up on TV shows and movies, which was fun after a week of starving, a reward for good behavior. When I was starving myself, I would have to keep busy; idle time was a recipe for disaster. Maybe I'd give in to the hunger and binge. Every day was the same—always busy, always tiring. When I was purging, I didn't have to work or work out—in fact, I didn't have to do a damn thing, because I was too sick and weak for the first twenty-four hours. I felt guilty letting myself relax normally. Normally, not being productive made me recoil like a gun accidentally firing in the wrong direction. But taking laxatives gave me an excuse to take the day off. The feelings of shame I associated with not doing anything didn't apply because I had to be near a toilet, which was actually productive; I was getting rid of calories, losing weight, and getting rid of the toxic "bad" foods I'd let into my body. Yes, I was in pain, and throwing my guts up was punishment, but it was my warped version of a vacation.

Movies were escapism. When I was watching them, I became engrossed in the lives of the characters and could forget about my own problems. I loved all kinds of movies, but my favorites were romantic comedies. I would root for the couple in the movie to wind up happy and together, and of course they would. In life, so many things are uncertain that rarely is there a completely happy ending. In the movies, chaos resolves. I was deeply comforted by their predictability and positivity.

The day following a binge, as punishment, I would not eat anything solid. Not even the one small diet microwaveable meal that became my daily intake. Saturday night, I would only allow myself liquid, a cup of chicken soup from a nearby deli to help the light-headed feeling pass. Relief would hit about an hour later when I'd look in the toilet and see the undigested pieces of carrots, celery, and parsley floating in the water, an indication that the food had not been digested. This assured me that everything I'd eaten the night before had been disposed of. By Sunday, I'd still be very weak and my stomach sore, but I would go in to the office, feeling nice and empty and ready to start the week off right.

On several occasions, I almost passed out after these laxative binges because I still had the responsibility of walking Teddy. Sometimes I would have to sit on the sidewalk and close my eyes, panting like the dog I was walking. I would take deep breaths in and out and wait for it to pass, thinking, *This isn't happening; please, whatever powerful force or god that is up in the sky watching over us, Care Bears even. Help me.* I'd sit in the elevator with Ted in my lap—I couldn't stand or I'd get dizzy again. That light-headed feeling—

where I should, in my mom's old song, sit and pause and "dingle dangle dingle" my legs to avoid passing out by getting up too fast— would creep up like a chill. With all my will, I'd fight the urge to faint. I knew if that happened, I'd wind up in the hospital, and then I would be discovered.

Eventually I would make it back from our walks, but I would feel so weak I'd drop to the first place I could—the carpeted floor, couch, bed, basically whatever could soften my landing. I would close my eyes and fall into a deep, cold, sweaty sleep.

There were times when Teddy would hold his pee for twelve hours because I was too sick from the aftermath of laxatives to walk him, which made me feel awful. We would just cuddle in my bed all day, in between my stumbling to the bathroom with either diarrhea or vomiting. After these episodes, I could hardly make it back to the bed. My eyes would be bright red and my body fragile. I'd take Teddy in my arms to make everything seem a little better.

"I am *so* sorry, Teddy. I am *so* fucked-up," I'd say. I deserved to self-destruct. I couldn't even take care of myself, let alone a dog. *You are completely worthless.*

I binged and purged this way from ages twenty-two to twenty-five. Even before this pattern began, years of throwing up had worn down my tooth enamel, and my back teeth were rotting. At age twenty, I'd had to get my teeth replaced.

"Do you have stomach problems?" the dentist had asked. "Or do you ever make yourself throw up?"

"No, me, make myself sick? NEVER."

"Well, it's unusual to see such terrible rotting for no reason."

"So weird," I replied, lying through my teeth (literally!).

Tooth replacement was so painful it would have made a normal dieter assess their behavior. But the thought of stopping never even crossed my distorted mind. That's how strong anorexia is; it is not a diet gone awry. It is an all-encompassing mental illness.

Now, at almost twenty-five and purging much worse than I had five years earlier, I began the fourth year of my spiral. My anorexia-bulimia combo morphed into full-blown anorexia. The practices were similar to what I'd been doing, but without the weekly binges and purges. During work, I would drink Diet Coke throughout the day to distract from my hunger. Between work tasks, I would maniacally research different diet microwaveable cuisines to see how many calories were in each. I started to like Garden Lites soufflés, which I often chose because they were extremely low in calories. I read that people ate it as a side dish or snack. It was my one and only meal of the day.

I would hang out in the grocery store for half an hour or more, comparing the calories in different packages, ranking them in my head from lowest to highest calorie content. I would usually purchase the one with the lowest calorie content, despite the many choices. I made sure there was no other food in my apartment, so I couldn't binge. This all may seem redundant, and *so* repetitive, but *that*, my friends, is addiction—and I was a food addict. And because of that, to me, it became a game, a hobby, an obsession.

I hadn't been on a vacation since I'd started working in the winter of 2008. So, in 2012, I agreed to take a full weekend off work to meet up with my parents, and my aunt, uncle, and younger cousins, at Disney World. Yes, the magical land of joy where there are *no* insects except for beautiful butterflies. I imagined the seven dwarfs sneaking out in the dead of night and killing all of the ants, moths, and spiders. Come on, there has to be an underground or dark side of Disney—where Mickey is smoking a joint, while Minnie is go-go dancing. *Nothing* is ever that perfect.

I was nervous about this trip and no, not because I couldn't trust those seven exterminating dwarfs. The truth was, I hadn't been around people during meals in a while. I had made my life so isolated that no one was ever around. How would I pull this trip off without being discovered? I wouldn't. It was impossible for me to disguise something that had become so visible and scary.

On our way out of the Magic Kingdom, my dad and I wanted to get gigantic stuffed animals for our employees to bring home for their grandkids and families. While my dad was paying for the Mickey Mouses, I walked outside the store to talk to my aunt, uncle, and cousins. Dylan, the older of my two little cousins, who stood about as tall as my hollow, bony chest, gave me a hug.

"Why are you so skinny?" she asked, without looking up, arms still wrapped around me.

I wasn't expecting that. I nervously twisted my curls, hoping an answer would come.

"Because she works out a lot and doesn't eat anything," answered my uncle for me. His words seemed to play in slow motion; especially the "doesn't eat anything." Yes, it was true, but hearing it out of someone else's mouth, out loud, made it that much worse. I wanted to cry. It just wasn't that simple, but I couldn't even explain myself. Even if I had something to say, which I didn't, my voice would be too shaky. I couldn't hold it together. I didn't want this.

My uncle is a broadly built man, a self-declared foodie whose wife is a pastry chef. They love food and so do their kids, and they could never grasp the concept of someone having such an aversion to it. Hence my uncle's seemingly insensitive words.

Dylan looked up at me, her arms still hugging, and said softly, "I wish I were as skinny as you."

Her green eyes were so soft and innocent. I didn't want them to be anywhere on me. I held my breath.

"No, Dylan, you don't want to be *anything* like me. Please don't ever say that. You're beautiful." My voice cracked as I fought the shame. I lifted her hands from around my waist and backed up, trying to create space between us, with the rationale that the farther away I got, the less she would want to be like me.

As I turned, I couldn't hold back my tears.

"Dani, what's wrong?" my mom said, coming out of the shop with my dad. She looked at me hard, concern in her hazel eyes. I shook my head; I didn't want to speak. My dad grabbed my hand and squeezed it hard in a way that meant, "I am here for you."

As we walked away, the tears continued rolling down my face, and my parents' comforting voices were muffled together in the background. I was a terrible example to any child. How would I ever be a mother one day? I wouldn't. I couldn't. Even if I hadn't destroyed my body already with the abuse I put it through and I physically could conceive, I just was unfit for motherhood. I was so ashamed. I never wanted anyone to want to be like me. Some people don't need children to be happy or feel fulfilled. But I'd always held out hope for motherhood. I am nurturing, that's why helping people is something I truly love—it's second nature. If I couldn't or shouldn't (meaning surrogacy and adoption would be out of the question as well) have children, I'd be losing the thing I most wanted from life. Motherhood was my only shot at happiness, and at this moment, I saw it as a clear impossibility. What, then, would be the point of living? Answer: there was none. The world and everyone in it were better off without me.

FULL LIFE, MAY 2013

My hands felt the room's walls as I walked in. It had changed a lot since I had last been here. Everything seemed smaller, my bed especially, even though I was living here only a couple of months ago. I remembered it being so big and comfy, and now it was small and kind of hard. I sat down on it, testing its bounce, picking up a brown teddy bear leaning against a pillow. It was wearing a yellow shirt that said "bee mine" above a little stitched bee. My dad had won it at a carnival for my mom when they were sixteen. They had a sickeningly cute love story—*The Notebook* level of adorable. It made me nauseated, but in a sweet, jealous way, not a gross, green, throw-up way. I put the brown bear down.

I picked up a gray bear from my bed. This one was in scrubs and a surgical mask. My grandpa had gotten it as a gift and given it to me, knowing my love for teddy bears. I, of course, didn't know it was a re-gift. It always meant so much to me because he gave it to me the last time I saw him before he passed away, when I was thirteen. I scanned all the bears on the bed. Every one of them had a meaning or a little story.

"Looking around?" My mom walked into the room, holding Teddy, and plopped on the bed with me.

"Yes. Just looking around, I guess," I said, biting my lip. "You know, Mom, none of this is your fault. I am not like this because of you guys. I had a great childhood, and I hope you don't blame yourselves." I placed my hand on hers.

"I know, but it feels good for you to say that. As parents, we tend to blame ourselves."

I thought about how this awful illness would affect my child if I had one someday. *What would I do? What could I do to protect my child? I would have to be in a good place myself. Would that ever happen?* I decided to write a post on my Living a FULL Life Facebook page:

Dear Future Child,

I will make sure you are protected to the best of my ability. I will be extra sensitive because I know there is a genetic component in eating disorders and you could be one of its victims because of me. I will never complain about my body in front of you. The words "fat" and "diet" will not be in our family's vocabulary. I will demonstrate a healthy lifestyle, so you can pick up on the idea of moderation. No matter what kind of day, we will always have dessert. I used to call dessert "berserk" when I was little. I couldn't say the word correctly. Oh irony! I think it's berserk not to eat dessert if you like it! Life is too short not to enjoy it while we are here. I will teach you that when you are being hard on yourself. I will teach you that bodies are vessels and what they do is much more important than what they look like. I will teach you that bodies come in all shapes and sizes and that's what makes them beautiful—how diverse they are. It scares me that I could give you this, but I know what to do and am FULLY prepared. I can't protect you from the world, but I will do my best. I will help form an army of mothers that can band together and fight society breeding future kids on the same path. You will help me choose recovery again and again, because I want to be better for you. I want this world to be better for you. I will fight, for you—because you will make everything worth it.

Love always,
Mommy

I pressed Post and sat back on my childhood bed. I pulled the covers over my shivering body. The house was freezing.

"Do you think I will be a good mom one day?" I asked Teddy. I knew I hadn't been the best mom to him because I was so messed-up, but that could change, right? I could be better. I was the best I could be...considering.

"You will be an amazing mom. You are going to beat this thing." I looked up and saw my mom's head peer into the room. She was just passing by. I smiled at her.

"Thanks, I love you, Mommy," I said, as she made her way toward her room. I wasn't sure if I would beat this; nothing seemed certain right now, but I was glad that she had faith in me.

"I love you too," she said. She had no idea how much her words meant to me.

Besides the obvious changes to my body—ribs jutting out of my torso, hips like knives—full-blown anorexia had other effects. My hair had started to thin out and become brittle. I had bald spots forming in patches on the back of my head, but I wasn't really self-conscious about it. In fact, I started not caring about my looks. I wanted to be invisible, and the uglier you are, the less you are noticed. Once, when I was getting my nails done, the manicurist asked if I was interested in waxing the hairs on my hands and knuckles. I looked down and noticed the light soft fur that had grown to keep my hands warm. I laughed and brushed it off as "always being like that," giggling because, shit, that was kind of embarrassing. I mean, move over Teen Wolf, this adult anorexic is the new werewolf in town. Sheesh. But in truth, I was so disconnected from my body, I had never seen that hair before.

My parents would often complain that my breath smelled like garlic, or comment that I needed to brush my teeth better; my mom was always pushing mints on me. "Hunger breath," which is caused by ketosis—a medical condition in which the body starts breaking down fat because the person is not consuming enough calories—is common in people with anorexia. Chewing food increases saliva in the mouth. When you are not eating, saliva decreases and bacteria growth increases, causing bad breath.[3] I was eating so little I most likely had a bacteria colony inhabiting my mouth. No matter how many pieces of gum I'd shove into my mouth, the stink would remain, because I wouldn't eat anything to get rid of it.

My mom would later mention the big circles under my eyes, clear indications of how sick I was. "The hollowness of your cheeks and those big dark circles," she would repeat, biting her lip and tearing up, as she talked about my descent toward death.

There is a myth about anorexia: that we look in the mirror and see a fat person no matter how skinny we are. Wrong! I knew how tiny I was, and I knew it didn't look good. Us anorexics, we aren't delusional, just sick. We see every hump in our spines. We see our arms and our legs becoming sticks. The problem is that we can't make ourselves eat.

In my opinion, my upper arms were the real giveaway that something was wrong, because they were thinner than my elbows. I had to cover them, especially during the summer season when I was expected to wear T-shirts, shorts, and the dreaded tank top.

I was cold all the time anyway. Even on a warm summer day, I would feel a chill down to my bones. In the winter, I would sit in my apartment in layers—two sweatshirts, one North Face winter coat, thick woolen socks, and sweatpants. I would top that off with a hat, scarf, and gloves and huddle in the living room under a soft blanket. I would still shiver. I dreamed of heat almost as much as I dreamed about food and calories, which is ironic because both heat and calories have energy, which I had none of.

My face had sunken in and turned yellowish, pale, and blotchy. It looked almost gothic. All I needed was black lipstick and I'd be set. In the shower, I would measure all the bruises. There were so many from walking into things at night when I was messed-up on pills and booze. So many black, blue, and green bruises, red marks, and scratches; a rainbow of self-hate.

> *Mirror, Mirror*
> *Why are you so cruel?*
> *I see bones,*
> *But all I can think about is fat.*
> *I can't look away.*
> *Why do you trap me?*
> *Why am I so sad all of the time?*
> *I can feel the end near.*
> *I can feel it in the dark undertones of my*

---

3   WebMD. "Oral Care/Bad or Changed Breath—Topic Overview." WebMD.com. Accessed August 22, 2016. http://www.webmd.com/oral-health/tc/bad-or-changed-breath-topic-overview

Beaten-down soul.
I won't have to be me anymore.
I won't have to live each day.
Trying to be everyone's perfect
And failing.
It's so hard.
It hurts everywhere.
Please go away, pain.
Maybe I will disappear.
I am almost there.
Mirror, you tell me that.
You never lie...

I developed recurrent corneal erosion syndrome (RCES). (I hadn't heard of it either.) One morning in September 2012, I woke up, eyes swollen and dripping, sensitive to light, one completely sealed shut by sleep crust. I pulled on it, trying to get it open, and screamed, causing Teddy to shake ferociously. That would be my first of many experiences like this. It usually occurs in people over forty. I was twenty-five.

RCES means repeated episodes of superficial spontaneous abrasions leading to eye pain. Erosions are "scratches" on the surface of the cornea. In many cases, the cells of the outer layer of the cornea are loosely attached to the underlying tissue. These cells spontaneously slough, leading to recurrent erosions.

> *"Patients typically present with attacks of mild to severe eye pain, redness, tearing, and light sensitivity. Some patients may report blurred vision. Most patients report symptoms after awakening from sleep."*[4]
> —Digital Journal of Ophthalmology

I would wake up almost every other day with an intense throbbing in one of my eyes, like salt being rubbed in an open wound. It made me afraid to go to sleep at night and more dependent than ever on the Xanax and alcohol to calm my nerves.

On the days when my eyes flared up, my face would be deformed from the swelling. I would lie on the floor at work in unbearable pain despite the dimmed lights. Looking at the computer burned, but how could I work without it? 95 percent of my day was spent staring at that screen. This was my livelihood, my adult responsibility. People depended on me. I needed to work through it.

I went to several eye doctors, and they hinted that my condition could be from lack of nutrition and dehydration, but I

---

4   Adamis, Anthony P., and Fina Cañas Barouch. "Recurrent Erosion Syndrome (RES)," djo.harvard.edu, October 15, 2002. Accessed August 22, 2016. http://www.djo.harvard.edu/site.php?url=/patients/pi/434

ignored their prompts for me to admit I was starving myself. When asked why I was losing weight so rapidly, I said it was because the problems with my eyes caused me so much pain that I couldn't eat. The erosions became my scapegoat. The fact that my body was falling apart was an excuse to fall apart more.

Around this time, nearing my twenty-sixth birthday, is when I became dangerously thin. At twenty-three I pulled off ninety pounds pretty well because I am petite, but now I was a good freshman fifteen less—a complete skeleton. Dr. Blatter, my therapist, had grown concerned and during one session, he finally voiced his worries.

"Dani, every time I see you, you seem to be getting thinner and thinner," he said, staring at me, looking at me hard, as if he were waiting for a response.

"Is that an observation or a question?" I cross-examined, shrugging so wildly, I knocked my special "dry-eye syndrome" glasses (that protected my eyes from light, wind, dirt, and debris) off my face.

"I thought maybe you would have an explanation. Have you noticed your weight loss?"

I shrugged again, saying nothing, bending over and grabbing my glasses off the floor.

"Okay, so you don't know why you are losing so much weight." He said, scribbling something down on his notepad.

"Well, my eyes haven't helped."

"Uh-huh, and anything else?"

I glared at him. This went on for the rest of the session. I sat there in complete silence as he asked question after question. I was irritated and afraid. *Was he going to hospitalize me? Call my parents?* I felt like he was accusing me of something, so I stayed silent. Or, in the words of my favorite talk show host, Andy Cohen, I pled the fifth.

My body had become so accustomed to starving that it didn't send me hunger pangs anymore. On laundry day, I could tell by the holes in the back of my sweatpants that cutting myself had become more frequent. Some holes were bigger than others, which indicated that I had managed to insert the knife into an existing hole without seeing it—an aptitude I hadn't aimed for, but was impressed by nonetheless. My sweatpants were a source of comfort, but also my measuring stick of how much weight I was losing. Afraid as ever of the scale and of the number it might read, I'd mark my weight loss by where the knife holes on my sweatpants sat on my body, slipping from their original position on my lower back to my tailbone to my butt, after which I would knot up my waistband to keep my comfortable companion from slipping to the ground.

One day, my doorman approached me on my way out and tapped me on the shoulder. I always walked with my head down, deep in thought, not paying attention to my whereabouts, so his tap startled me, so much so that I tripped over my own feet, luckily catching myself before I fell to the ground.

"Dani, are you okay?" he asked.

"Yes, I wasn't paying attention. I am such a klutz, but I caught myself—"

"No, are you *okay*? You've lost a lot of weight recently," he clarified. He had a look of genuine concern. His face was squinting, revealing soft wrinkles on his forehead. I saw that his jet-black hair had wisps of gray growing in.

"Yes, I am fine," I said, through gritted teeth and continued out the door. Me—the girl who was described as "too sweet and nice" in her sleepaway camp days and probably most of her life, an empath to the T—was now unrecognizable. Did I have PMS? No, I hadn't menstruated in over a year. I was far too skinny for my body to actually work. I was tired of everyone commenting on my weight. Why couldn't they mind their own business? I had not lost a lot of weight recently. I looked the same. *Yeah right. Even you aren't that delusional.*

The fact was, I was almost disappearing, and I liked the idea of that more than anything. I couldn't live the way I was living anymore, like this—it was exhausting. Like Princess Aurora of *Sleeping-Beauty*-narcoleptic-spell-bound fame, I needed a long, drawn-out sleep. Goodnight world.

> *Mirror, Mirror on the wall*
> *Who is this person judging me?*
> *Gazing, with her skin and bones.*
> *Tears in her hollow eye sockets*
> *Red and wounded*
> *Ribs protruding outwards*
> *Cheeks gone*
> *Who is this person?*
> *She isn't a person*
> *She is a ghost*
> *She is unrecognizable*
> *She is the voice's creation.*
> *She is anorexia.*

My OCD grew manic, and I became paranoid. At night, I would open and close the closet door, repeating, "I wish I was the skinniest person in the world and the prettiest person in the world." If

I didn't say these words, I would gain weight or find myself bingeing uncontrollably. I just knew it. Then I would go to the front door of my apartment and check again that it was locked. Then to the second bedroom to turn the elliptical on and off, to make sure it was working. I didn't want it to be dead if I tried to use it. Because it ran on electricity and was plugged into the wall, that thinking didn't make sense, but none of my thinking did. Then I would run to the couch where my knife was waiting and place it on my back and sit on it, letting it rip through my skin, calming me.

If I felt uncomfortable, I would repeat this pattern, again and again. I would inspect every crevice of the apartment, checking for hiding trespassers, one of my greatest fears. It was as if I believed ninjas were after me, using cameras to spy on my behaviors, waiting to expose me. I'd check under the bed, in the closets, behind the shower curtains, and so on. *If anyone saw my behaviors, I'd be hospitalized, or worse, institutionalized.* By the time I sat down for good, I felt dizzy from all of the exertion. I would drink my wine and take my Xanax and slowly calm down, drifting off. I was absorbed in my self-destruction, stuck in the hell in my head.

Drinking, drinking myself half to death, like a fish. Drinking to numb out and finally pass out, insomnia free—peace. Drinking to not think about food, calories, body image-any of it.

Mix of alcohol and prescription pills makes me paranoid before bedtime. No time to count sheep—no time to jump over the fence and follow the herd—one, two, three. I duck and look under beds—in closets, cabinets, searching like Sherlock Holmes. For who? Anyone who is going to bust me—imaginary handcuffs around my wrists. Anyone who is an undercover spy, going to report me to the "anorexia police." I routinely check around my apartment until I black out. No more paranoia. No more awake life, just darkness.

I wake up on the couch, floor, and bed if I am lucky, eyes crusted over and head splitting into two.

There are moments when I get terrified and cry my head off. I want to run away. I can't live like this anymore. Where to? Anywhere. Just away from my mind. My face crinkled from stress like worn leather, horror in my deep brown eyes. I am driving through a dark hole fast; my body can't keep up with my brain. Nothing is in my rearview mirror except for sadness and bones, stacks of both.

I can't stop. I falsely believe drinking brings me closer to the gray area. The area that seems so far far away like my very own unattainable Neverland. Fly, fly like Wendy, Peter Pan and Tinkerbell. To a place where everything seems more hopeful, magic is plentiful, and food isn't Captain Hook.

There were the forgotten years. Those years lost in black outs, calories, OCD repetition. The years that all blend together—masked by darkness.

One day I will awake and realize all these behaviors are self-destructive. Band-Aids on a deep dark wound. That is the day I will start seeing Neverland. Through a light in a long-tired tunnel, I will see it.

I imagine in recovery, I am there. My gray area is found. I let myself feel. Pain, pleasure—all of it. I am living. I am as real as the Velveteen rabbit. Loved from the inside out. I am free from anorexia's web. I am FULL.

November 2012 was my cousin's wedding. It would be my first public event in a *long* time. I wouldn't have done this for just anyone, but I adore my cousin. A dutiful bridesmaid, I complied with the bride's insistence on my wearing a strapless dress. My arms were on show for all to see. My collarbones protruded from the low-cut dress. I could feel the cold air touch my exposed spine, and I shivered. This dress was the tightest piece of clothing I had worn in many years, and it made my body stiffen in discomfort. Its purple hue clashed with my yellow-white skin. It was not a good look.

I had begged my mom to get me a shawl, and she'd had one made out of the dress fabric, so I would feel more comfortable during the reception. However, I would have to walk down the aisle without it—thanks, bridezilla uniform!

When the big day came, I didn't eat breakfast and lied about lunch as the other bridesmaids munched on mini-sandwiches and drank champagne, without a care in the world besides stray hairs in their updos—priorities, people. Thank goodness for hair spray—phew. I got my hair done while chatting with my other cousin, the bride's older sister. She confided that she was pregnant, touching her still flat-as-a-pancake stomach. I jumped up and down with excitement. That was the first time I had smiled with genuine happiness in a long time. While we got ready, we took photos, the flashes hurting my sensitive eyes. I snagged a drink here and there to get me through.

When the time came to walk down the aisle without my shawl, I was tired from standing for so long and my feet hurt from my high heels. I was not good at walking in general, but heels were like putting stilts on an elephant.

I was paired with my older cousin's husband, who was instructed to slow me down because I have a tendency to walk too fast when I get nervous. Walking down the aisle, I kept my eyes focused straight ahead, imagining being at my own funeral, with an organ dirge playing in the background. It was the only way I could get through it, thinking this was the last time I would see any of these people anyway. The unfortunate side effect of the leisurely pace was that it made me acutely aware of all the eyes staring at me. And the shocked whispers were hard to ignore—Dani looks terrible, my aunt's friend hissed, craning her neck to get a better look. I will be gone soon.

The ceremony began, and as I saw the love that the bride and groom had for each other, I started to cry. My habitual numbness lifted, and suddenly I was feeling everything. I cried for how beautiful their love was and for the endless possibilities for their future family. And I cried because I was well aware that I would never have that kind of love or future.

They kissed, solidifying their union, the crowd giving a standing ovation, and we headed to the cocktail hour, where I grabbed my shawl and wrapped it around my bony shoulders. Much better. During the wedding festivities, I hung out with my great-uncle at the bar. He is of Irish descent and could drink with the best of them, and one thing you know about me at this point is that I could too. Especially when I was in a social situation that involved food— bring on the vodka!

"Dani, I just...I just really wish you would be easier on yourself," said my great-uncle. "You are such a good person and have so much going for you. It's hard to watch you like this." He was wearing a tuxedo, and his Anderson Cooper white hair was slicked back just like the silver fox himself. He took a swig of his Grey Goose on the rocks.

"Thanks, Lar, don't worry, I am good," I said, voice wobbling. I began playing with the long hair extensions that I'd put in for the wedding. They made my face look less gaunt and hid my bald spot.

We drank and talked at the bar, watching people on the dance floor shaking and jiggling their hips to the music. The bride was in the middle, center of attention, in all her glory, beaming.

A little while later, walking to the bathroom, I came across a childhood friend's father, a doctor.

"It is so good seeing you," he said, embracing me—I could feel his warmth against my cold skin.

"You too," I answered, voice flat, knowing the hug was unavoidable. It was over before I could stop it.

I wasn't open to hugs because I was afraid someone would feel my bones. They would know I was not okay by how delicate I felt. I could usually disguise it in layers. Not today. Sometimes I imagined someone squeezing me so hard I would snap in half. Put me, snap, right out of my misery. But I was a little drunk and my reaction was delayed, so I welcomed the hug with open arms.

Usually my reluctance was paranoia, but this time my hugging hesitation was spot-on. I later found out that he was scared for me and told my aunt to talk to my mom, that I needed serious help. I was a shell of my former self and so close to death's door. I knew it, he knew it, and I was at peace with that.

While people all around me were living, moving on, building lives, enjoying one another, I waited for death. I thought everyone would be better off. I thought I would be a burden, especially if I got the help I needed. Every day was so hard. I had given up on myself without even *really* trying to get better. My behaviors were so entrenched that, in my mind, I was the problem. ED and I weren't two separate entities. We were one really messed-up person who couldn't be saved.

Weddings were bad news, but at least they were rare. Holidays were the bane of my existence, and when you're Jewish there are a *lot* of them—all with elaborate dinners. We Jews love food. I mean, in a culture where chicken noodle soup is penicillin, what can you expect? That year, 2012, I opted out of all holidays, even Thanksgiving.

Holidays are the worst when you have an active eating disorder. Everyone is there, analyzing what you look like and what you put in your mouth. It is neither relaxing nor fun to be around all that food, especially when the eaters are commenting on how "fattening" it all is and how they'll put on their "fat pants" and diet tomorrow. *They expected me to eat all that fattening food after that?*

People who meant well would patronize me with exaggerated displays of enjoyment: "Mmmm, Dan, you have to try these mashed potatoes; they are *so* delicious."

With each bite everyone took, with each bite I took, with each moment where I felt abnormal, the feeling that I couldn't go on escalated.

Day after day, weekend after weekend, were the same. Saturday and Sunday, I would usually sleep in, then go in to work for the latter part of the day, to keep myself busy and resist the urge to binge followed by the urge to purge. Alone at night, I'd chase Xanax with alcohol and then eventually pass out a la Lindsay Lohan circa '07—in the front seat of a car, mouth wide open, eyes sealed shut— just subtract the car and add a couch and bingo, that was me.

Then, one Sunday morning in December, just a month after my cousin's wedding, I woke up on the couch in the living room, Teddy sitting on my chest and staring at me bug-eyed. I petted him and looked at the clock. The lights flashed eight a.m., making me fully aware of my hangover, and I needed Advil like five minutes ago. I had a free day ahead of me, no obligations. I could wake up and go in to work, but then I would be done around one, because I didn't have a full day's worth of work on a weekend. What would I do after that? I couldn't volunteer anymore. I was far too sick and weak to partake in the one thing I loved. I had become a burden, even when trying to help others (a.k.a. taking-the-last-cup-gate at the shelter). I didn't have any friends left in my life. I let them go and they stopped trying after a few times of me bailing on plans. I was too caught up in my illness to think clearly—believing they didn't care about me. In my mind, no one did. They would all be better off without me. I also couldn't sleep any longer—I felt annoyingly wide-awake. I picked up Ted and juggled him from hand to hand.

"What to do, what to do," I said, continuing my little game of toss with him. Suddenly, my stomach gave an involuntary lurch—*growl*.

"Ah, Ted, and now I am hungry," I said, giving him my best pouty face. I got up, leaving him on the couch, and looked out the window. It was pouring outside, the kind of day where you just want to stay inside and hide under the covers with a handsome lover, but I didn't have one of those either. I couldn't just rest here and not work or volunteer. If I were sick, I would be allowed to sleep and watch movies all day. I could also fill this growling tummy, taunting my fat ass. This seemed like a no-brainer. Movies, sleep, and purging it was.

I grabbed my iPad and quickly, before I could have a chance to second-guess my decision, ordered a cinnamon raisin bagel with fat-free cream cheese and a fat-free muffin. That would seem like a normal breakfast to most, but I would need a side of seventy-five Dulcolax to get rid of it—like the way a Big Mac goes with a side of fries. Dani *actually* eating went with a side of laxatives. Because I hadn't been using laxatives much in the past year and was subsisting only on one small microwaveable meal a day, my body didn't need the usual 150–175 to get the job done. This was my new "binge and purge lite."

I counted out the pills, one by one, and placed them on my living room table. Then I swallowed them one at a time as I waited for my food to arrive. The tiny orange pills worked better on me than any other laxative, and they were easy to get down. Between pills, I looked out the window as the rain kept drip-dropping on the windowpanes. Teddy had fallen asleep next to me. His black-and-white fur was moving up and down mechanically as he breathed, as if he was battery-operated.

The doorbell rang. I answered and grabbed the bag, ripping it open in anticipation, my stomach growling fiercely. I gobbled every morsel of that delivery and then got into bed and fell asleep for a couple of hours. Nausea woke me up, and I knelt over the toilet on the bathroom floor like the old pro I had become.

Throwing up, hacking so terribly that it scratched my throat, was followed by a terrible cramping. Since I hadn't purged in so long, the aching in my gut was extra intense, a sick, stabbing pain. The sweat beading on my face puddled on the cold tiles as I lay on the bathroom floor. My vision started going in and out.

I could hear my mom singing the dingle dangle dingle song. The thought of her soft voice comforted me. Shit, I had to get up off the floor; diarrhea. I put my hand on the bathroom sink to pull myself up. Then I sat on the toilet to an explosion-like sound, a war of sorts, headed from my body into the toilet. The pain was so bad. To comfort myself I found myself singing.

"It's time to dingle dangle dingle

It's time to dingle dangle dingle"

My eyes closed, I bit my lip. I wiped and flushed the toilet. I put my body back on the cold floor to rest. I continued faintly:

"It's time to dingle dangle dingle

Dingle dangle time."

This was the end. I could feel it in how my body was breaking down and reacting to the laxatives. I imagined my mom and dad coming into the bathroom and finding me dead. I could see my mom shaking me, tears pouring down her face. I could see my dad calling 911 and embracing my mom, holding her tight, just as scared as she was. Their lives would never be the same. They would be the couple that discovered their dead daughter on the bathroom floor of her apartment. I would want to hold my mom's hand and tell her, "You think you are sad now, but if you knew the real me, you wouldn't want me to live either," but I couldn't because I would be dead, gone, in the ground. I repeated these words out loud: "Dead, gone, in the ground."

With that thought, I drifted off. Every time I woke, Teddy was there. I'd pet him or give him an encouraging glance. The whole day and night, I lay there with intervals of horrible diarrhea. I felt weak, faint, and every move was hard to make. That whole day was a blur. I looked over at my phone, and it had a text from my mom that said, "Good night, Babyface. I love you."

My cell phone showed 2:45 a.m. when I wrote back, "I love you too." I was going to die today. I was seeing things—me, in the desert, vultures circling overhead. Then I would come to—me, on the tile floor, eyes blinking, vision in and out. What was real? But I'd miss my mom and dad if I were dead, and what would happen to Teddy?

What if I got help? *No!* It was like I was tossing a coin: on one side was life, the other, death. *But what if? No!* Back to the vultures, circling and circling, getting lower. I sat like this, tossing this imaginary coin from hand to hand. I was either all in or all out. One minute I was all in, the next I was all out, vultures closing in. Finally, I was—

All in.

At five in the morning on Monday, December 3, 2012, I texted my mom, "I need help."

My mom and dad didn't even ask what that meant. They knew. They rushed into the city as soon as I sent the text; it was as if they had been waiting for it. They had, in fact, been waiting for it. For years.

I was crying hysterically. I knew I was going to be sent away to a hospital or a treatment center, but I assumed that was the only way I could get better. I was exhilarated, but terrified. It was what I imagine jumping out of a plane must feel like. I was jumping into the unknown, free-falling into this world of recovery.

How long would I be sent away for? Where would I go? As I started packing, I looked over at Ted. How could I leave him? How could I leave my whole life? But I had to do it.

With that thought, my mom and dad barged into my apartment. They threw a bunch of clothes and Teddy's things into a big red Kipling suitcase that, to my delight, still had the little gorilla dangling from it. In all this chaos, I was able to smile because of it— because it was cute, and because I was so afraid.

My mom and I discussed that I would probably only need comfortable clothes wherever I was going. Repeat: *wherever I was going.* My mom threw leggings, sweatpants, long shirts, and sneakers into the bag. I couldn't even help, I was so numb and afraid. Had I made the right decision? What was I getting myself into, with no possibility of turning back?

I picked Teddy up and we all headed out, locking up my apartment for what I knew would be a while, not sure if I would *ever* be back.

In the car to my parents' house, I left a message for Dr. Blatter on his machine, asking about treatment options. I needed his professional opinion, even though he's not an eating disorder specialist. We all did. Safe from myself at my parents' house, I finally got some sleep. I drifted off only to wake hoping it was all a bad dream. Unfortunately, it was about ten in the morning and I was *still* at my parents' house. I tried pinching myself awake from this nightmare. *Damn it, still here.* I pinched again. *Ouch.*

What was going on at work? My dad had left for the office shortly after we got to my parents' house. I would be missing a Monday at work to rest and to figure out where I was going to be shipped off to. *Bon voyage, Dani.* How scary! I never missed a Monday, and it irked me, especially knowing I would be absent from a big board meeting. My new reality was that I was going to be missing a lot of Mondays. Trying to come to terms with that gave me incredible anxiety, like a scratching-my-skin-until-it-bleeds level of anxiety.

Meanwhile, I kept getting sick to my stomach from the laxatives, the remnants of what I was hoping would be my last purge. After all, my eating disorder had accompanied me for over a decade and a half. I deserved freedom from its web of restrictions. If only I could get rid of it using a vacuum, duster, or bleach and water, like we did on those pesky spider webs that loomed in the basement of my parents' house.

With that thought, I went downstairs to the kitchen to find my mom (after all, she's the spider web removal expert). She greeted me with her eyes, but there was no smile. She wanted answers. At her insistence that I explain my bad stomach, I disclosed that I'd taken laxatives. I even disclosed how many. As she put her hand over her mouth, horrified, I thought, *if she only knew how many I usually took.*

We were in our usual seats, where we would get into cereal fights, laughing late at night, but now the mood was somber and scary. My mom insisted on making me a turkey sandwich on whole-wheat bread to coat my stomach. I hesitantly agreed. "I need to take it slowly," I told her. She sighed. She equated getting better with gaining weight, which she would soon learn was not the whole picture. To her, food was medicine, and she needed to feed her dying daughter to save her.

My anxiety increased as I heard Mom move around the kitchen, opening drawers, closing cabinets. I didn't look, but I knew what she was making, and that I'd be expected to eat, so each drawer slam made me flinch, as "turkey sandwich time" got closer. As she placed the sandwich in front of me, I began to calculate calories. I couldn't shut it off. One slice of turkey deli meat was about 29 calories; she put three on the bread, which was 87. One slice of whole-wheat bread was 69; there were two slices, which added up to 138. Altogether, 225 calories, give or take.

As I took the first bite, my hands started shaking. I thought about all the calories flowing through my body, and it wasn't even eleven o'clock! I had a whole day of eating ahead of me! It was so hard to even chew and swallow; my whole body was shaking like crazy, rejecting the sandwich. I took a deep breath and sat back. Something wasn't right. My head felt light, but different from the feeling when I was going to faint; it was a scary and unfamiliar feeling. I looked over at my mom, and then, like magic, everything faded to complete darkness.

HISTORY AND PHYSICAL

NAME: SHERMAN, DANIELLE

DATE: 12/3/12

HISTORY OF PRESENT ILLNESS: The patient is a twenty-five-year-old female with a long history of eating disorders, anorexia and bulimia, who presented to the emergency room after she sustained two episodes of weakness and seizure. She has not been eating for a while and took a number of laxative pills yesterday and today she had a turkey sandwich at parents' home and right away, had a syncopal episode with a tonic colonic activity, first witnessed by mother and then by EMS. She is now alert, awake, and oriented x 3, and there were no prior episodes. The patient has been working with a psychiatrist and was supposed to go to rehab tomorrow.

PHYSICAL EXAMINATION:

GENERAL: She appears in mild distress secondary to anxiety and appears cachectic.

VITAL SIGNS: Blood pressure is 94/50, heart rate is 69, temperature 97.2 degrees. Her weight is 36 kg with BMI of 15.

HEENT: Exam shows no scleral icterus. Somewhat dry mucous membranes.

Dressed in only a thin white gown, I shivered ferociously under the plush white blanket my mother had brought from home. I couldn't move, not even to make eye contact with my mother, who, flanked by doctors and nurses, peered over me.

"What happened to me?" I wanted to ask, but I was too confused to form words. My head hurt. I closed my eyes to relieve the pain and blurriness. I could hear the wails of the ambulance, so loud yet ever fading as I went in and out of consciousness.

"Danielle, can you hear me?" the EMT asked, with such command it scared me into answering him. But what came out of my mouth was only gibberish, like a record played backward in slow motion. The one thing in English I could say became my mother's saving grace as she squeezed my hand in terror: "I don't want to die."

My abuse of laxatives had been going on for a good ten years, and I was finally paying the price. I'd thought I could feel my body breaking down the night before, and I was right. I had known something bad was going to happen, and it did. Like I had a crystal ball, I'd predicted it, and I was lucky I'd asked for help and wasn't alone.

I noticed myself drifting off and quickly opened my eyes. Something else would happen to me if I let myself relax. I didn't know how stable I was. I heard a rustling at the side of my bed and jumped a little.

"What are you doing here?" I asked, finally able to get some words out, when I saw my dad kneeling at my bedside. The ambulance had safely landed me in the hospital, where I'd been put on an IV while unconscious. "What about your big meet—"

I had convinced myself that no one cared about me to the point that I couldn't believe he was there.

"No meeting, nothing, Dani, is more important than you." He grabbed my hand, and I squeezed his to try to comfort him and let him know I was going to be okay. I wasn't sure I was, though.

According to my mom, I had fallen sideways off the kitchen chair and begun shaking rapidly and uncontrollably, my body alternately contracting and relaxing. She'd pinned me down, like a wrestler, so I would stop shaking, then immediately dialed 911. The doctor and EMTs said I'd had a seizure.

The MRI revealed nothing unusual, and considering my weight and past history, the theory was that my low weight put me at risk for a seizure; the relentless diarrhea and vomiting induced by the seventy-five laxative pills I'd swallowed the day before were enough to get the job done.

This was the longest day of my life. It was like a complex jigsaw puzzle; I couldn't solve it, to get the full picture of the day. All I really remember from the hospital is my exit that night—the only thing I didn't selectively block out. I couldn't wait to get home, back to Teddy, and out of this scary dream-like reality.

The seizures had turned my legs into lead, making it impossible to walk. My whole body felt limp as my parents wheeled me out in a wheelchair to Dad's car. Was this a test to show me how important my body is? The voice in my head screamed, *You should have tossed the coin the other way. Death would have been so much easier. You are hopeless.* What would be next? I couldn't imagine staying there, in a hospital. Was that where they were going to send me?

When we got home, my dad carried me up the stairs and placed me on my parents' comfy bed. I was spoon-fed egg drop soup by my mom because even my arms were too stiff to move. With each spoonful of salty egg drop in my mouth, I realized I had lost all independence. I was being fed like a six-month-old. I was even going to sleep with my mom tonight, and something about that made me feel safe. I wanted her close by, and I could tell she wanted to be near me, too. By the time I closed my eyes, it felt so good to let myself relax. I weighed seventy-nine pounds. I was exhausted.

PART TWO

Full

CHAPTER 10
The Lone Naked Tree

I woke early the next day. I had an appointment with Evelyn Attia, MD, director of the Columbia Center for Eating Disorders, at eight in the morning. I had firmly decided the night before that I would try to get better at home by participating in an outpatient program while continuing to work. I had convinced myself that, if I went away, my dad would find someone better, smarter, prettier, *anything*, and replace me. I was also terrified. I had always imagined residential treatment to be like sleepaway camp from hell, filled with spiritual bullshit and fattening food. I also felt like I needed to have some kind of independence and focus outside of my recovery, and work would give me that. I couldn't just leave all of my responsibilities behind me, Teddy included. I mean, I could if I really had to, but I didn't want to. This was my final decision, and I stood firm on it, like a contestant confidently locking in their "final answer" on *Who Wants to Be a Millionaire?*

We drove to the city, to the Upper West Side. It was freezing, and I was bundled in a scarf, like a cloth shield, but could still see my breath in the cold winter air. Snow covered the streets and grounds of Central Park West in a glittering blanket. The scene was breathtaking. I hadn't taken a real look around me in a while. On the side of the street, there was a sloppy snowman gleaming from his sheen of ice, bent down as if greeting cars that passed. His nose was a crooked carrot, eyes chocolate chip cookies, mouth a Twizzler smile. *What a fattening, gluttonous snowman.* The trees were contrasting, bare-naked, with only snow covering their knobby branches. I couldn't help but feel like one of those naked trees, stuck in the ground, leaves and everything gone, nothing left to give, skinny, cold, and alone.

I could still see my breath as we walked into the ornate pre-World-War-II building. I pushed a button and a buzz let us in.

"Well, here-eee..." I paused, then tried again. "Here we are." I laughed at my stutter, trying to lighten the mood and interrupt the deafening silence. It was still hard for me to talk, and I was forgetting words often. The doctor said this was normal after a seizure, but language would come back. *Gosh, it better. I didn't think it was possible for you to get more stupid. Of course, you'd find a way, Dani.*

I sat down in the waiting room. Across from me was a tiny wooden table holding magazines—I bet there were no health, fitness or fashion magazines. Underneath was a deep blue carpet that covered the whole room. I tapped my foot impatiently on it as I debated getting a magazine, more so because I was curious to see if my prediction was right.

My parents sat next to me as I switched from foot tapping to playing with my itchy red sweater, which covered my black tights down to my knees. I kept the green scarf-shield around my thin neck. My mom had pulled it around me this morning when we were getting dressed—another layer that made me look less sick and helped keep my body insulated. She also blew my hair out strategically to cover my bald spot, topping my look off with blush on my pale face to "give me some color." I wanted to give this prestigious doctor a good first impression. My life was in her hands, as much as I hated to admit it.

I crossed my legs and tried to sit up straighter.

Before I could move to get a magazine, this woman who was going to determine my fate was standing right in front of me. She had short hair and a really strong handshake, which told me she was confident and competent right off the bat.

As we followed Dr. Attia, I spotted my arch-nemesis standing in the corner of her bathroom: the scale. I eyed it as we entered her office; I had radar for scales and was hoping she wouldn't make me get on it. She sat the three of us down on a couch and smiled at me, motioning for me to come with her. We walked out of her office and into the bathroom where she gently closed the door behind us to give us some privacy. It was just the two of us—and that damn scale giving me the stare-down.

"I am going to weigh you," she said calmly. "I would prefer you didn't know your weight, so we are going to have you stand backward on the sca—"

"Good," I interrupted, knowing where she was going with this. "I really don't want to know my weight and how much I gain either."

"Okay, good," she said, and had me turn around. I saw her jot down some notes in a notebook.

I got off the scale and followed her back into her office. She shut the door and sat down. While we were making introductions, I expressed my plan of going into an outpatient program while continuing to work. While I was in the middle of making my case, Dr. Attia cut me off.

"I'm afraid you are too skinny and sick for an outpatient program," she explained. *Shut down.* "In fact," she continued, "it would be detrimental to the patients to see you there in group therapy, because they are much further along in recovery than you." *Ouch.*

"What are her options then?" My dad asked, giving my hand a supportive squeeze. "This choice is not up to Dani. We need to do what gets her well and that is up to you. She is our life, so our lives are in your hands." I squeezed his hand back because he was so sweet, not because I agreed with what he was saying. Hell no, I didn't.

"Well, because her weight is so low, her options are hospitalization and residential treatment. She needs to be in an around-the-clock program."

The words "No outpatient," "residential," and "hospitalization" all stuck like peanut butter to the roof of my mouth.

"There's one more option up for consideration," Dr. Attia told us. "We can try the Maudsley approach."

Bless you, I wanted to say, because it sounded like a sneeze. We had never heard of anything like it.

I was excited to learn that it was an alternative to being sent away. I was willing to do anything, *anything*, to stay away from what I pictured as anorexia hell—complete with devils (scales) and perpetual torment (being force-fed copious amounts of food).

As we learned, the Maudsley approach ("weight restoration") is an intensive outpatient treatment where parents play an active and positive role in order to: (1) help restore their child's weight to normal levels, (2) hand the control over eating back to the adolescent, and (3) encourage normal adolescent development through an in-depth discussion of these crucial developmental issues as they pertain to their child. Maudsley considers the parents to be a resource and an essential component in successful treatment for anorexia nervosa. Basically, the parents are responsible for feeding the child and finding any acceptable way to be sure she eats. The parents are full members of the treatment process and an integral part of recovery. There would, of course, be modifications based on my age. I was an adult, so these standard rules would be customized to my needs, and not being an adolescent would make this a trial of sorts.[5]

The perception of the anorexic being a teenager is a myth. Women of any age can adopt disordered eating patterns to gain a sense of mastery over stressful situations. Part of my embarrassment about asking for help was that I'd always thought I was too old to still have my eating disorder. I should have beaten this years ago, nipped

5 Le Grange, Daniel, and James Lock. "Family-based Treatment of Adolescent Anorexia Nervosa: The Maudsley Approach," Maudsleyparents.org. Accessed August 22, 2016. http://www.maudsleyparents.org/whatismaudsley.html

it in the bud—which, of course, made me more of a failure. But this was simply not true. Though teens and young adults are more likely to experience anorexia or bulimia, moms, dads, and older women and men are at risk as well. Also, I am far from the first person to have a chronic secretive decades-long struggle with anorexia/bulimia that went untreated until adulthood.

"So, what is Dani going to work on with you?" my dad asked, never one to be shy or wait to be addressed.

Dr. Attia crossed her hands in her lap as she spoke. "Various things. I can tell you generally. When we briefly spoke on the phone, you were talking about Danielle's eating patterns, and I understood about her very rigid eating and things had to be just so and structured a certain way and there was a lot that was secretive about it for her. You told me about all of that. A lot of it will be my educating Danielle, and she has her therapist (I had agreed to go back to Dr. Blatter again). She has someone else to support her, so we will mainly be discussing what is hard about making change and what could be dangerous about not making change as far as this eating disorder is concerned."

I held on to those last words, drifting off in thought. "Change." That word always scared me. I was well aware of everything that was at risk. It was going to be hard for me to be okay, and even though I wanted to get better, a part of me was afraid and unsure that I *really* could. I'd only gotten the extra push to get help because I'd found myself in a health crisis. If I hadn't had the seizure, I could have backed out. I had backed out before. But this time was different. Staying ill, now that everyone knew, now that I had verbally committed to recovery, wasn't an acceptable option. Now I couldn't back out.

Dr. Attia's voice came back into focus as she looked past me, at my parents. "The seizure really helped mobilize what was going on. It was frightening to everybody, which allowed you to do what is very hard in an eating disorder, which is to say, *I can never put myself in that situation again. What other options are available?*" Her eyes scanned the room again, and then they rested on me. "What are you most nervous about, now that you are about to embark on recovery?"

"I am anxious about my weight changing and getting fat. I really want to push through and just get there, but I am afraid I won't be able to."

"When I work with people, I tell them some version of 'Fake it till you make it.' It's some version of let's just do it, and if you hate it, we can go backward, but what if it's not so bad when you get there? I always do a lot of encouraging, even on the short term—just try it, just try it, just try it."

Dr. Attia directed her attention to all three of us and continued, "I mean, what I am asking you to do, it's terrible. I am asking you to do something that your brain is totally against, and you luckily have things that are motivating you for you. You have just been through this scary time; you have your parents really articulating why it is important. You have a lot that is driving you toward health. But you have this illness that also comes with the little voice up here," she said, pointing to her forehead, "that says, *Don't do it, or don't do it so fast, or don't do it this way. Don't do it just because she says so.* It's an illness that comes with a voice. None of that is pleasant."

"Yes, none of it is. If I can be open and honest with you, I am actually really embarrassed because I don't consider myself a superficial person." It felt so good to openly talk about this. "I think I was ashamed for so long because I am not that person who cares about these kinds of things, but at the same time, I did! I mean I hate shopping, I am not into stuff, and I could wear the same comfy pajamas everywhere every day and be happy, and then I was so obsessed with being thin because it was the only thing that made me feel better. Yet it came off so shallow and made me hate myself for being so surface."

"There is nothing to be embarrassed of," Dr. Attia assured me. "This is a disease, an illness, like cancer. But you brought up a really interesting distinction, and that is one of the challenges in the treatment. You can feel like 'I hate this person who has become so obsessed with something superficial like being thin, I hate myself.' Sometimes, that self-hate drives more of these wacky eating-disordered behaviors. Yet, I don't think that person you have grown to hate is really you—that is this illness. You look like all the other people with the illness, but of course you can't be like all of those other people. Every person is an individual, but that distinction is so hard to make when you are in it."

"Yeah, it makes you feel worse about yourself. I mean, I hated myself so much for what I became," I said, looking at my parents. This all seemed new to them, and they were quiet, which was very out of character for them, especially my dad.

"Of course, it makes you feel terrible!" Dr. Attia exclaimed.

"It's like a self-fulfilling prophecy."

"Of course it is, and while I am going to ask you to increase your eating and increase your weight along the way, this illness is going to make you feel worse, not better, about that. Then you will be there eating and possibly gaining weight, but feeling so awful about yourself, so your instinct will be to go in reverse, to try to lose a little more weight because maybe you won't feel worse; maybe you will feel a little better, but of course what happens? You feel worse. It's really hard, and you are going to have a lot of challenges, but I know you can do it."

"Thank you," I said, leaning back further on her big black couch. It was relieving to have someone know my disease so well. It almost made me feel normal.

"Do you know which DSM-5 category you would categorize her as?" my mom asked, obviously having done her research on eating disorders. She was referring to the *Diagnostic and Statistical Manual of Mental Disorders*, fifth edition, a diagnostic tool used by the American Psychological Association.

"She meets anorexia nervosa DSM-4 and DSM-5. It's called binge-purge subtype because of her laxative abuse."

"It is interesting, though, because no one knew she had a problem until she was at such a low weight that it became obvious to the naked eye. We didn't really know about the laxatives until we found them. It's so easy to hide these eating issues," my mom mused. "Is it common for people to vacillate between anorexia and bulimia?"

Dr. Attia settled back in her chair. "Let's say a few things about this: It is not entirely uncommon for eating disorders to migrate from one category to another, so a lot of people may start with some restriction and wind up being called anorexia nervosa, but maybe they can't restrict or don't restrict, and then there is binge eating, and their weight maybe moves up to a different category, and then the name of what they are struggling with changes. They may have bulimia and they may have binge eating, if that's what happens."

"If you have eating disorder behaviors for a longer period of time, is that when you start going back and forth?" my mom asked curiously.

"Yes, with early intervention, people are sort of identified earlier, so they haven't had it for that long. If that's the case, the prognosis is much better. It probably just means that the behaviors aren't so entrenched. It can become more entrenched if you have the illness longer, but I never give up. I have seen people who have been ill sometimes for decades and decades and decades, and then something clicks for them. They really want to make a change, and they get there. There is nothing about anyone's story that ever makes me give up."

"That makes me feel better," I interrupted.

Dr. Attia smiled, and then continued speaking to my mom. "We are going to treat her for anorexia, though—not her bulimia. When we say *anorexia* and *bulimia*, in the current way we describe things, we separate them. It really can't be that you have both at the same time. If you are low weight, so many things are going on with you medically. Your treatment and your illness and your risks and your everything are so determined by being in that category that we called it *that* category—whether there is purging or there isn't purging, it doesn't matter. Anorexia is what it is, and the treatment needs to be like the treatments for anorexia. If people are normal or above-normal weight and consume large amounts of food and compensate by purging or other versions of those behaviors, we put that in a different category. It's more in the bulimia-like category, and the treatments that work tend to be the treatments that help in bulimia. These are different from the treatments that work for anorexia. So we tend to separate the groups out. It's not like everyone flip-flops and goes into different categories. It's not like you have to spend your whole life at the edge of your seat, saying, 'Oh my God, when is my next phase of an eating disorder going to develop?'"

"Have you ever treated anyone else her age with the Maudsley approach?" my dad asked, wanting to know her qualifications and if this *really* was going to work. He was hoping with all his might that eating disorder recovery worked depending on the doctor's success rate, like a brain surgeon's.

"Not so much with people her age," said Dr. Attia. "I've treated people who were a little younger than her with Maudsley, but I haven't treated young adults with Maudsley. It seems perfect for this situation though, because," she looked at me, "you really don't want to go to the hospital."

"I really don't!" I agreed.

"And you're close to your parents, plus you share an office at work with your father. So this combination makes it really worth trying." Her eyes moved from me to my parents. "Some of the groups that developed Maudsley started to study young adults, but I have never done that work before. I have been trained in Maudsley very specifically. I just thought if she is really going to try to avoid structured treatment programs, and she is going to stay at work, she needs helpers."

"And we are more than willing to be those helpers," my dad said, satisfied with her answer.

So: My parents were going to be in charge of preparing my meals and making sure I ate each bite. I would not be allowed to exercise or move back to my apartment in the city or have other adult freedoms until I hit certain weight-gain milestones, which I wouldn't be privy to.

I would also see Dr. Blatter twice a week and Dr. Attia twice a week, where I would be weighed, and we would talk about the process, emotions, food, and so on. Once in a while, we would have a family session with Dr. Attia. I would also be required to keep a food journal to record how I was feeling during each meal and talk about the whole process (for an in-depth look at this four-month period please refer to the Food & Feelings Journal in back matter). Additionally, I agreed to go on antidepressants to help with my depression and anxiety. If I wasn't making progress with my weight gain, I would be sent to a hospital or residential program, no ifs, ands, or buts—as in, my ass would be sent to anorexia recovery sleep-away camp hell A-stat.

My parents agreed, and so did I. With a handshake, our team agreement was sealed. I was no longer alone. It was no longer solely anorexia and me. I was going to bloom into a beautiful tree FULL of leaves, not the lone naked twig I had become.

CHAPTER 11
Maudsley

People deal with things in different ways. My dad's attitude about my eating disorder was: *Let's fix this right now. Let's make her okay. Let's shake her. Let's scream at her. Let's intimidate this eating disorder out of her.* He would get frustrated and yell, "Why can't you just take care of yourself and eat?" I couldn't. When I slipped with laxatives during my time at home, he thought I was being deceitful. It wasn't me. It was my disease, my addiction; it was a brain pattern that I could not control—autonomic synapse firing patterns that were embedded after a lifetime of these behaviors. These coping mechanisms were no longer a choice. I wish they were.

My mom was more understanding and sensitive about the process. She understood that I was very sick. She was nervous and would blame herself, which was rough because it was not her fault.

The process wore heavily on both of my parents. It is not easy on anyone when one member of the family isn't well, especially when the disease is so elusive. My mother and father stuck by me, but living with my parents, having them controlling my every action, especially my food intake, was not easy. It wore heavily on me.

My birthday was December 19, sixteen days after my seizure. Normally I didn't do anything. I despised the attention. I was like the Grinch of my own birthdays, even hating balloons because of the sound they made when they popped. But this year would be different.

I cried. Yes, I was reduced to pathetic tears of self-pity. My eyes and face were a salty, snotty mess, as I lay in a pile of wet tissues.

"Dan, stop feeling sorry for yourself. This will all get better," my mother said, trying to make me laugh by putting Teddy in my face and doing her best Teddy voice, if he spoke English and could sing "Happy Birthday."

"Come on, Mom, let me feel sorry for myself. By the way, you are losing your mind." I pulled a pillow over my head to absorb tears that continued to flow.

Doesn't she get it? I hate where I am in my life. I can't believe I'm twenty-six years old, basically ordered to live back at home or else be sent away to a hospital. I'd be better off dead. My sobs turned to wails as my mother rubbed my back, like she'd done when I was little. Happy Birthday to me.

✕

Even though I was gaining the weight—the scale said it and, trust me, I felt it—my eating-disorder thoughts weren't rapidly dissipating. In fact, at times they felt extra strong. One of the theories of Maudsley is you need to first feed the brain, so the chemical imbalances correct themselves, making it possible to begin recovery. I didn't feel that happening. I was just gaining the weight and still felt absolutely miserable most of the time. Even more miserable because I was being forced to eat, and the antidepressants I'd started taking for my depression and anxiety weren't going to work until I was back to a normal weight. Starvation affects the function of neurotransmitters in the brain, making antidepressants ineffective.

The initial physical weight gain was tough to take in. I quickly found out when I started gaining the weight that my stomach would grow round and out, swelling like I was a starving child in a UNICEF commercial. Panicked, I called Dr. Attia, who confirmed that this was a common side effect of long-term malnutrition and it would eventually normalize. All I could hear was *eventually*. As I continued to gain, the fat distribution was also very uneven, as my body, which still thought it was going to starve, attempted to hold onto nutrients for dear life. For someone with anorexia, weight gain is hard enough, but weight gain coming in like this took my living hell to another level. I had to avoid mirrors because it became that much harder to face the next meal. I also found that, every time I attempted to eat, my body would shake, sometimes so hard I could hardly put said food into my mouth, because I was so nervous about what I was about to do. I still had guilt related to the food because, unfortunately, anorexia was still very much looming. It was very hard to push forward and through these obstacles and bad feelings.

During this time, I read an article on *Psychology Today* online titled, "Starvation study shows that recovery from anorexia is possible only by regaining weight." One paragraph really stood out to me.

> *There is no point in waiting for the magical moment at which you decide, once and for all, that you want to start eating more again, or to regain weight. Your starved state is making you unable to think flexibly enough to FULLY comprehend the possibility of eating or living differently, or even the possibility of wanting to think about and enjoy things other than food; it has hidden*

from you who you really are, and made you believe
you are nothing but the anorexia; it is making
the smallest piece of food feel like too much.
For these reasons you will never truly want to
recover, but you have to seize all your feelings
of despair, desperation, hope, recklessness, and
curiosity in order to make yourself plunge into
that first day and first meal of recovery. As long
as you keep yourself going, keep eating, through
the first difficult weeks, it will get easier and
easier. [6]

Even though I'd hit rock bottom, I would never be totally ready to get better. I had to just keep on eating, like *Finding Nemo's* Dory just kept swimming. She eventually found her way, and so would I. Trying to get through each meal, especially in the first couple of weeks, was the hardest thing I ever had to do in my entire life. I would have to believe that when my BMI was eventually normalized and enough time passed, my mind and body would be at peace. So I just had to keep pushing through, despite everything in me wanting to fall back on my old ways. This didn't stop the eating disorder voice from battling me at most meals.

One day, I couldn't take it anymore. I sat in front of my food and hesitated. Something possessed me. "I hate you and I hope you *die!*" I screamed at my mom. I wanted her to tell me that I was the piece of shit I knew I was. I wanted her to say she didn't care about me and I was a waste of her time. That would be my excuse to self-hate, not care to recover anymore, self-destruct. I wanted to hear it. I wanted the permission to give up on myself. If only she would first.

She snapped. She took me to the back door and threw me outside as I screamed louder and louder: "I hate you, I hate you, I HATE YOU!" Then she pulled me back in, as if she'd had a sudden change of heart, and she hugged me.

She realized it wasn't me screaming. It was the anorexia that hated being fed. She began to cry, and I did too.

"I am so sorry. I just don't think I can do this," I said, weeping, my head in my hands.

"Yes, you can, Dan. It is going to be okay. I love you." She stroked my tousled brown curls slowly. She took a deep breath and

6   Emily T. Troscianko. "Starvation study shows that recovery from anorexia is possible only by regaining weight." https://www.psychologytoday.com, November 23, 2010. Accessed August 25, 2016. https://www.psychologytoday.com/blog/hunger-artist/201011/starvation-study-shows-recovery-anorexia-is-possible-only-regaining-weight

paused for a moment. We both took in the silence, our thoughts filling it enough, until she spat out, "Don't do that to me anymore."

"I won't." I promised, between slowing-down sobs.

"You were pretty scary. You looked like you were possessed," my mom admitted, her hands shaking a little.

"I think I was." I laughed, my voice still quivering.

We both began laughing because we were done crying and there was nothing else we could do. From then on, she would call anorexia "the devil inside of me." And it was.

Then there were the two relapses. The first was during stage one of Maudsley, where my parents were controlling every morsel of food I put into my mouth.

Empty, empty, empty, I wanted to feel empty. Lighter. So I bought and abused Colace stool softener, thinking I wasn't *totally* breaking the rules if I bought something I was allowed to have in the first place, since my mom gave me two pills each morning. I was taking twenty a day, to be precise. And I got caught.

My father and I were in the car on the way to work when my mom called.

"Do you have something to tell me?" She was eerily calm on the other end of the phone.

"No, what are you talking about?" I hissed, annoyed by her accusation, lying to myself and knowing I'd fucked up badly. *What does she know? Shit. I know what she knows.* I looked at my dad. He was on his cell phone, oblivious.

"Dani, I am not mad."

My eyes welled with tears; my worst fear had come true. I had been caught. "I am so, so sorry," I said, clenching my jaw. I hung up the phone and looked at my dad again. My dad looked at me but didn't press. "I think I need to go home," I told him. He nodded, knowing if I needed to miss work, something pressing was going on.

We were already near the George Washington Bridge, and he had to be at work early for a meeting, so he dropped me off at a Starbucks in Fort Lee in a strip mall near the bridge. I waited anxiously for my mom to pick me up, holding onto each second of being alone, of not having to explain my actions. I thought about going to the nearby CVS and buying more laxatives, since my mom had discovered my only stash. *Shit, who thinks like that? I am such a fuck-up.*

I sat in Starbucks with freezing cold tears rolling down my face. I was exhausted—sick of this entire draining process. Should I get a tall hot tea to warm my hands? No. I couldn't be trusted doing anything right now. The addiction was so strong, I might run and buy laxatives at CVS instead of going to the Starbucks line. People kept coming in and going out, getting coffee, living normal lives, and I was envious of each one of them. I tried to hide my head with the hood of my jacket, so nobody could see my red, tear-filled face. That's the point of being so thin; you can disappear and hide.

After what seemed like a long fifteen minutes, my phone rang.

"I am right outside," said my mom. I didn't reply. I just hung up the phone and took a deep breath.

I went toward the car, hesitantly opening the passenger door of the white Mercedes. I got in, ready to be scolded, but my mom surprised me with a hug. She felt sorry for me, and so did I. Her hug felt warm and inviting, comforting. I cried on her shoulder as she held me. We remained like that for a couple of long minutes, not saying anything. We didn't need to.

Though I already knew what this was about, my mom revealed that she'd found the bottle of Colace hidden beneath papers in a bottom drawer in the computer room. This obviously wasn't a surprise for me, because I put them there. She explained that she'd found it odd that I had been going into that room so often over the past couple of days. Sometimes, even when I knew she was around, I had such a strong urge to take them that I would risk getting caught and go get them anyway. I mostly snuck down there in the middle of the night when my parents were sleeping. I was ashamed. I had compartmentalized it in my head as *not a slip*. Otherwise, I was doing so well—eating, and gaining weight.

"I need to call Dr. Attia. I don't know how she will want us to handle this."

"Fine," I huffed between sobs, embarrassed. *Oh no, not Attia. It made my failure so much more real to have the doctor know about it.*

Dr. Attia assured us it was completely normal and a small setback. She said we would just have to rebuild from here. Start over. She was so calm because relapse is so common in recovery that it is actually one of the steps of change.

The stages of change are ambivalence, contemplative, pre-contemplative, planning, action, and maintenance/relapse. Relapse is a step because it is natural for it to happen; you just have to be willing to admit it and go forward. It is completely normal to go backward, once you've moved forward, in the stages of change. I was still in the early stages of recovery, and that's why I think I was more upset about getting caught than I was about committing the crime.

She also spoke to me briefly, and I could still hear her encouraging voice on the phone hours later: "This is an illness. Sometimes this illness is going to poke its head out and be active. You have to call me at these times."

I would have to get to a point where I wanted to be stopped. Where I valued myself enough to not think of myself as a bother or burden by doing so. I'd vowed to get there. One day...

My other relapse was during the second phase of Maudsley, where I was taking back control over my eating. By this point, I'd gotten back some of my privileges by reaching weight milestones. I was able to participate in yoga, eat alone if I had to, choose my own foods (my parents having veto power), and was getting closer to the desired twenty-pound-plus weight gain. I was looking stronger, but I was still struggling mentally with my changing body and eating through the changes. This relapse caused a much worse reaction than the first one, because my parents felt more betrayed this time around. They were further invested in my recovery and had put more trust in me, and then I did this...

A couple of weeks after the first laxative incident, my mom found natural laxatives I'd bought in one of the drawers in the computer room—a different drawer; at least I was smart enough (debatably) to do that. I had once again compartmentalized the laxatives as not being a problem. They were.

I had again tried to justify them to myself because they were "natural" laxatives. *Natural* meant they were acceptable in my mind. My mom called my dad when we were on the way home from work and angrily told him what she'd discovered. He yelled at me for being deceitful.

"All you do is lie to me. I can't fucking trust you! How could you lie to me?" he roared, his lower teeth overtaking his upper lip like a Shih Tzu, which was intimidating as fuck—not like the cute little Shih Tzus I was familiar with.

"I am so sorry, I didn't mean to—" I said, biting my lip hard, tears in my shame-filled eyes.

"You mean, you didn't mean to get caught! Your mother and I have been busting our asses trying to get you better, and this is how you repay us. You are so ungrateful."

He had such force in his voice that the car shook with its booming vibrato. He never knew how to handle his emotions, especially over things he couldn't control. He didn't understand how powerful this addiction was. He didn't understand that the last thing I wanted to do was lie to him, to my mom. It wasn't about trust. I had a problem. I was an addict.

I cried all the way home as he expressed his disappointment in me as a person, and even more hurtful, as his daughter. We got home, and as we pulled in, I saw the outline of my mom at the door peering out: her long brown locks, medium-height lanky body, and long skinny arms. How would I get around her without talking to her?

I opened the car door and slithered out like a rattlesnake making its escape, slammed the door shut behind me, and ran past my mom up the back stairs and hid. Yes, you read that correctly, *I hid*, like a little girl avoiding her spanking. Through the vents, I could hear them talking, but only in murmurs. Then they shouted for me: "Dani! Dani!" I stayed in my hiding spot, paralyzed.

I hid in a closet in my room, under hanging clothes, squishing old shoes with my butt and legs, for what seemed like a long time. I whimpered but tried to stay as quiet as possible. It was hot and dark, with a little light peeking under the door. I saw the backs of dresses from when I was younger. One was dark maroon. The dress I wore to my bat mitzvah. I felt the texture; hard, almost stale. Over my head was the suitcase where I used to hide laxatives; now I was hiding because of them. I'd reached a new low.

"Dani, Dani! Is this a joke? Where are you?" I heard my mom's faint footsteps far away.

"Did she leave the house?" asked my dad.

I heard the front door open and slam shut.

Tucked quietly away, I let them panic. I let them squirm the way I had been squirming these past couple of months, tiptoeing around them, trying everything to please them, following their every fucking order so I wouldn't be hospitalized. I resented my dad's reaction; I resented my mom for busting me the way she did. She could have just waited until we both got home, instead of making me get stuck in a car with someone who saw this as *the ultimate betrayal*.

"You are going to be in big fucking trouble whenever you come out!" I heard my dad scream. Not exactly motivation for me to move. I closed my eyes and tried to slow my breathing, hoping the walls of the closet would close in and suffocate me, end it all right now, right here.

"Dani, please, we are not mad at you," my mom countered his lunacy. Her panicked voice made me feel a little bad.

About ten minutes later, I opened the closet door from the inside, revealing myself. I picked myself up slowly, feeling weak and defeated as I called out, "I'm here, I'm here." But my voice was a whisper, not the shout I'd intended. "I'm here. I am coming!" I called again, this time louder.

I walked down the front stairs and found them both in the kitchen.

When I saw their faces, I apologized through broken whimpers and tears. My parents both embraced me. I snuggled into my dad's chest, hiding my face and tears in the warmth of his body. I cried for my parents. I cried for myself. I cried because I didn't think I could do this anymore. I just cried.

Maudsley is an intricate and intimate process, based on unconditional love and trust in each other as a family unit. What results is far more than recovery—it is a closeness and richness in relationships that becomes a gift, a silver lining for a very dark cloud. My family and I are all better people because we shared this process together.

I would say to any parent of a child with an eating disorder, "Don't blame yourself; don't blame the child. You are all victims of this disease. If you stick together, you can break it." And that's what we planned to do.

CHAPTER 12
Gradual Reentry

The pattern went like this: My parents would scrutinize something I ate or didn't eat, I would get upset and throw a fit like a moody teenager—*I hate my life, you guys don't know how hard this is,* etc.—and then my mom would comfort me. I couldn't live like that anymore. I just needed them to hear me out. Old Dani wouldn't tell them how she felt. New Dani realized she had to stand up for herself in life and couldn't hold things in that were bothering her or she would self-destruct. I had to make some necessary survival decisions, or the three of us were soon going to be reenacting a battle scene out of *Lord of the Flies.* Plus, I am pretty sure I would play the role of good-natured Simon, and he died, so things would be looking pretty grim for me in combat.

I decided to have a rational talk with my parents.

"Look, I know this hasn't been easy," I began, nervously twiddling my thumbs, "but I need you to trust me. I know it's been tough for you guys, but it has been the hardest thing I have ever done." I paused, gathering my thoughts. "What I am trying to say is that refeeding alone is hard enough, so we really need to find peace between all of us if I am going to continue spending so much time with the both of you. Correction, I mean *all* of my time." *I needed to get to the point.* "I am doing well and need both of you to recognize that fact. Maybe loosen my leash a little. Please." *There.*

Silence. I looked down at my feet, trying to avoid eye contact while no one was talking.

"We are going to try to start trusting you more with eating, but we are nervous," my mom finally said, looking at my dad for backup. He nodded, following my mom's lead, as always.

They agreed: What a surprise! And I could certainly understand their hesitation, considering my relapses.

"It has been hard for us with you living here, too, under these circumstances, and at your age, after you have become accustomed to being on your own. You aren't the best at taking direction anymore," my mom added.

Well, I am an adult being treated like a two-year-old, I wanted to say.

"I know and understand," is what I did say. And I *did* understand. I felt like such a burden being there, on top of them, in *their* space, cramping *their* style every second of *their* day. Plus, I was a very needy houseguest/borderline prisoner at the moment. They both needed space from me. I needed space from me, so trust me, I understood.

Thank God, I wasn't going to have to live with my parents forever! We all decided—Dr. Attia, Dr. Blatter, my parents, and I—that I'd move back into my apartment in stages.

When the time I was so desperately waiting for finally came, I wasn't quite as excited as I thought I'd be, to say the least. I was actually reluctant, even sad.

I was not moving back permanently. I'd be half at my parents' home and half at my apartment, and being in and out like that seemed a little odd and uncertain to me—and by now, you know how much I *love* uncertainty. Also, doing anything halfway was, to me, a "failure." I didn't want to be back and forth, living out of a suitcase. My black-and-white, all-or-nothing mindset was still learning about that middle ground people call the "gray area."

I was so nervous that I might fall back. I stalled, using different excuses to stay longer with my parents.

"Oh, Dad is going to be away on business, so that's not a good night. I'll keep you company, Mom."

"Hmm, I think we have yoga that night, and I don't want to miss it."

"I think that night may be hard to pick up Teddy after work."

But eventually I realized I never would be fully ready, so I would have to force myself, kind of like that article in *Psychology Today* said about the whole refeeding process. Shortly after that realization, in mid-March, it happened.

Opening the front door, I jiggled my keys together; my hands shaking from nerves. I knew I was opening the door to a new life, and I was terrified of what that life would bring. The door eased open, and I wasn't sure if I should walk in. The apartment was pitch black. I turned on the light to a clean but empty apartment—naked and alone, like the twig I once was. I was so focused on my self-destruction, I hadn't filled the apartment with pictures, mementos, plants, anything. I walked into a blank space.

The first thing I did was go to my closet, or "hiding spot." I'd hidden my stash of laxatives in a brown boyfriend bag on a top shelf, under other strategically placed bags and clothes. I had too much temptation when I passed the neighboring Duane Reade and CVS; I didn't need more in my apartment. As I unzipped the bag and peered inside, I finally understood the phrase "curiosity killed the cat." *Dani, just one purge left; it won't hurt you,* called the pills. But a new recovery voice prompted: *This curious cat was almost roadkill because of you.* I had three boxes of 150-count Dulcolax and one package of ex-lax chocolate laxatives, a combo that guaranteed I'd throw my guts up. These would be very useful if I had a slip and binged. *One time wouldn't hurt me,* said the old voice as my hand shook, making the bag sway, whacking my leg as if encouraging me. *Yes, it will!* I countered, hurrying the bag to the garbage chute down the hall, where I tossed it and watched it disappear for good.

"Goodbye, past life," I said, wiping sweat off my face before closing the latch. With a boom that made me recoil—almost stepping on Teddy, who had followed me outside, as if saying he supported my decision—I said goodbye to my past. That bag had followed me to college, to both apartments, and now it was gone. I was no longer as sick as my secrets, because with those laxatives down the chute, I had nothing to hide. I was free.

I needed to start fresh and fill this apartment with only good memories going forward. I was going to become a beautiful tree FULL of leaves. I was determined. And I'd have to fill this place accordingly, make it more me, whatever that was.

This transition included many visits home for backup. One night, I was struggling with my self-esteem and began feeling sad. A glass of wine, and that sad feeling was five times more potent. *Binge and purge. Fill that empty void,* yelled the old voice. Grabbing my coat and Ted, I called a car service to my parents' house. They were going out for dinner with friends, but I knew being alone for the whole night couldn't be an option. So I went over to their house anyway; they would be back later.

Knowing that I was accountable to someone other than myself made me feel more confident that I wouldn't slip. It's funny how things had changed. I used to hate being around people, because that meant I had to eat. Now, I hated being alone because I was afraid I'd be pulled toward the empty—not eating, or abusing food and purging.

Overall, it was nice to have my space back. I had good days, okay days, and terrible days, but I didn't revert back to my old habits. It wasn't like I could snap my fingers and everything would get better all at once. Gosh, I wished it would be as easy as *Bewitched's* Samantha twitching her nose—and magic—voila, all better! But I was conscious enough now—self-aware enough—not to let myself fall.

After my move, my mom and dad began to get their lives back. As they planned for a two-week vacation at the end of April for my dad's birthday, I felt frightened. I would be alone again. I didn't want to tell them I was afraid, or they would cancel their trip. I needed to get a life of my own, so I wouldn't be so dependent on them. I needed replacements for my codependent relationship with anorexia. So the search began. My first stop: *a social life*.

I decided to start by contacting some old friends. I'd pushed a lot of people away during my four-year spiral. The first person I called was my friend Courtney. We decided to meet for dinner at a small sushi restaurant on the Lower East Side.

Courtney was the only friend who had reached out to me in the months leading up to my seizure. She used to invite me to Zog kickball, a program that gets people together to play a sport and go out drinking afterward. The lure for me was that the money we spent went to a charity of the winning team's choosing. I once went to kickball, but I didn't have enough strength to keep up. Skeletons don't kick very far. The former "soccer star" could hardly kick the ball past the pitcher, and me running to first base was probably a worse sight.

I hadn't seen Courtney since I had entered Recovery World, which resembled the dark side of Disney World that I had imagined, minus the characters doing naughty things to keep things interesting. Gosh, if only I could have smoked a joint with Mickey Mouse. Recovery World was a chaotic, dark world where you feel everything because you aren't allowed to numb out. It's terribly scary, like haunted-mansion-creepy-jumpy status all the time. But I digress.

I saw Courtney walk into the restaurant. She is model-tall and lanky, with long dirty-blond hair and deep blue eyes. She's fun and vivacious, with an always-interesting social life—think Carrie Bradshaw on *Sex and the City*. We have the shared history of being friends since the awkward days of middle school. She was a member of the popular crowd, so we didn't hang out as much on the weekends in high school, but we always remained close. She came over and embraced me in a warm hug.

"Hi, stranger!" I said, hugging back.

We sat down, and I adjusted in my seat, while she checked her phone and smiled.

"So what's new with you?" I asked, giving her a wide grin, knowing by that cat-that-ate-the-canary smile on her face, it must have been a text from a boy she was interested in.

"Well, I am kind of seeing this guy and…" She chatted on, telling me all about this advertising executive she'd met at a party. Her life seemed so *disgustingly* normal.

As she talked, I became preoccupied with my own insecurities. *I don't have much in common with anyone anymore. While she was being normal, with twenty-something boy troubles, I was living at home being force-fed. Who would relate to that?* Her normalcy was a breath of fresh air to my fucked-up existence, yet it also made me feel sorry for myself. I didn't tell her what I was going through. I was still too ashamed. I was like a mime, using gesture, expression, and movement during her stories, because I had nothing to contribute.

Shortly after that, I went out with another group of friends from high school and felt even more out of place. We met for dinner—Italian—but I couldn't connect with them. Since we'd last seen each other, they had all made history, formed closer bonds. I was the outsider, unable to contribute to the conversation because I had no idea what was going on. I was filler, that random friend they once knew—and that hurt. Because of my stranger status, I didn't feel safe. *Anorexia, where are you to comfort me? You* know *me*. Later, they would be in each other's bridal parties at their respective weddings. If anorexia hadn't created this gap, if it didn't haunt me, maybe I'd be there too.

After dinner, we went to a trendy lounge to meet up with their other friends from college. As we walked in, I admired the flashing lights filling the room like a 1970s disco: red, purple, green, blue. I was introduced to a handful of people. There was a preppy couple in matching polo shirts, two manicured blondes, and a few chiseled-jaw, master-of-the-universe finance types. Standing on the outside of the circle, listening to them whine about their annoying other friends in their social group, felt like hearing dispatches from a distant planet, a planet where I wasn't sure I was welcome or wanted to be.

"Hi, how are you?" I said to the girl in the polo shirt, her pearls matching her toothy white smile.

"Ohhh, hi, I am Robin. Nice to meet you." She said, as she gave me a manicured hand.

I had met her several times before. She was one of those people who pretended each time we came across each other that it was our first meeting. She was too important to remember me. Or maybe she had some weird form of early onset Alzheimer's but I think it's more of a life sentence of bitchery complete with resting bitch face!

"I am doing the paleo diet and lost five pounds already," she said, addressing the crowd. "It is perfect for your wedding, Britt! Your bridesmaid dress is going to fit me like a glove." Robin wiggled and did a little turn, showing off her five-pounds-lighter frame.

I kept a fake smile plastered on my face as I ordered another drink. *Vodka on the rocks, please. And make it extra strong.*

At one time, I had been very close with the bride-to-be, Brittany. But I wasn't invited to her wedding. We had been in touch throughout college; I had gone to her small birthday dinners up until the previous two years, when I was very sick. She showed me a picture of herself posing in her off-white Versace wedding dress, hand on hip, smiling wide.

I took her iPhone and looked at the picture. "Aww, Britt, you look absolutely stunning."

"Thanks," she said. "Want to see the bridesmaids' dresses too? Lindsey tried hers on today."

"Yes, of course," I said. Really, I couldn't have felt more left out, more unimportant, looking at bridesmaids' dress pictures for a wedding I wasn't invited to. I know it wasn't Britt's intention—she was just excited about her wedding, and not thinking—but, in that moment, I felt like I didn't matter to anyone but my parents.

When I went back to my apartment that night, I drunkenly examined myself in the mirror. I felt fat and horrible. I put my fingers over my belly, feeling the fat. During my time in treatment with Maudsley, I was told to process how I felt after I ate, and sometimes I would find myself jotting down *I feel fat*. Dr. Attia would counter that fat is not a feeling—angry, sad, mad—these are all feelings—and there had to be another word besides *fat* that I really felt.

Well, I never really agreed with that because, "You see, Dr. Attia, 'fat' is a feeling. Look, I can feel it now," I said out loud, cinching my stomach bulge in my hand and wobbling it around in the mirror. *Disgusting.*

For the first time since my second relapse, I had thoughts about laxatives. I couldn't tell my parents because they would freak out. I couldn't tell anyone.

I took my medication and got into bed, tossing and turning. *Where did I belong?*

The next day, my parents came into the city and forced me out of bed. My mom literally came into my bedroom, opened all the windows, and tossed the blanket off the bed, leaving me exposed to the blasting air in my apartment. In the words of Stephanie Tanner, *How rude!* With the lights blaring in my eyes and freezing cold air attacking my body, I had no choice but to get up. Gosh, I needed sunglasses and maybe more alcohol? Damn you, hangover headache. I blamed me, such an odd-man-out. That feeling drove me to the drink. *Ugh.*

"Mom, just let me take a hot shower and brush my teeth."

"Fine, but you have to get up. I didn't like how you sounded on the phone." She said while opening the blinds.

"You are killing my vampire status today," I moaned. "I am going into the shower. I'll be ready in fifteen minutes, stop opening things. I promise I am getting ready."

"Good," she said and shut the door to let me do my thing.

I felt a lot better once I got up. It would be good for me to go outside, even though my depression was pulling me toward the bed like a magnet to a metal fridge. Depression mixed with a hangover— not a great getting-out-of-bed formula. But it was nice having my parents with me for the day, having company, my support.

The rebuilding process was hard. When I started to come back to my old life, no one was waiting for me, greeting me at the proverbial door. Life had gone on while I was sick, and I wasn't even a thought after years of no contact. People changed, and so did I. But now was my chance to find people I really belonged with as "recovery Dani." Now was my chance to start over as a healthier version of myself.

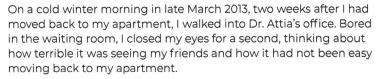

On a cold winter morning in late March 2013, two weeks after I had moved back to my apartment, I walked into Dr. Attia's office. Bored in the waiting room, I closed my eyes for a second, thinking about how terrible it was seeing my friends and how it had not been easy moving back to my apartment.

My thoughts were interrupted by the thump of a door shutting, making me jump. A tall, thin, beautiful blonde woman came out of Dr. Attia's office and scurried through the waiting room. Her dark blue eyes met mine, and quickly refocused on the floor. *She must have an issue as well, and she is not a teen, either. I am not alone.* As crazy and naive as this sounds, when you have an eating disorder, you think you are the only person in the world going through it. It's a very isolating disease, so there is comfort in that moment when you realize there are others like you—like this woman. *I shared her shame.*

I heard the rustling of papers and then in came Dr. Attia. She was wearing a bulky sweater and a long black skirt. "Dani, I am ready," I heard in echoes, as if she were far away. I secretly wished she were.

I silently walked into her office. I had been there countless times, almost four months of sessions, but still Dr. Attia intimidated me. Let's be honest: she scared the living crap out of me—like, I didn't need to take laxatives after a binge around her (too soon?). It was her tough demeanor, coupled with the fact that I respected her and didn't want to disappoint her. It was also because she held my life in her hands.

"How are you doing?" I asked. I felt almost claustrophobic from unease. I noticed that my voice was a little scratchy from the cold. I was debating about asking for water, but decided against it, thinking she would accuse me of "water loading"—drinking water to add weight before a session.

"Good, good. Take off your shoes, it's time for your weight," she said, getting up from her seat and heading to the scale. She always got straight to business.

"Yeah, yeah, I know the routine," I wanted to say, but I was too frightened to show any bit of humor, wit, or sarcasm, and quietly followed her to the bathroom.

She then patted me down to see if I was hiding anything anywhere to make me weigh more. I would later hear about people putting weights in their pockets or wearing heavier jewelry to weigh more. I wasn't crafty enough to think of those things, though, plus, I really did want to get better, despite my slips. On the scale, I faced in the opposite direction so that I wouldn't see my weight—the stipulation Dr. Attia and I had agreed to in the beginning, but that I had grown to regret.

I would often find myself eager to know where I was, number-wise, and afraid that I might be weighing too much for my standards, but Dr. Attia had promised me that she would let me know when I was one hundred pounds, and as of this session, I was not there yet. She said that I was close, though, and that both pleased me and freaked me out. I also didn't trust her completely. Correction: my anorexia kept me from trusting her completely. *How can I trust her? What if I am more than one hundred pounds, and she is lying to me? Let's not forget, this woman is the one who is trying to make me fat!*

She scribbled something in her notebook, and then she silently followed me back to her office, shutting the door behind me. I sat down on her black couch as she positioned herself cross-legged at her desk.

She didn't hold back. "You lost four pounds in one week."

I did? How is that even possible? I have been eating.

"Four pounds?" I repeated. I thought for a second. "I had my period last week, and didn't you say that I could be up in weight only because of that?" *I don't get why, when I gained weight last week, I was told that it could have only been because of my period. Now when I lost that water weight this week, it wasn't because I was fluctuating back to how I normally am.*

Dr. Attia ignored my point. She had no time for my excuses. "If you don't gain the weight back, we are going to have to move you back home or into a hospital, and you wouldn't like that, *would you?*" I figured that was a rhetorical question. Of course I didn't want to go to a hospital. Who in their right mind would want that? Especially after all the hard work and progress I had been making so far. I hated these scare tactics.

I felt a tear boil in my right eye and then my left. Damn copycat eye—hold out, lefty! No, now both are starting! I had cried about a million times in the past couple of months of us seeing each other, but now, as I felt it happening again, I wanted so badly to be strong. I didn't want to cry more than *anything,* even more than being force-fed something fattening with no nutritional value, like a donut. Okay, maybe not *that* much. But I was getting better. I deserved a chance. *Don't I? It is just a small setback, if anything at all, right?* Great—one million and one, here we go for the kill— and with that, the expected weather of precipitation down my face increased to 100 percent as the tears turned into a torrential downpour. I placed my hands strategically over my eyes, catching them before they made their way down.

I will always be grateful for Dr. Attia; she saved my life, and I will never forget that. But after that meeting, I decided that I was done with all this emphasis on weight and food, hospitals, and all this "hard love" negative crap. I was over writing about it and talking about it. It still made it all such a focus in my life, and I didn't think that was healthy. This negative focus was getting depressing. It was hard enough to rebuild my life as it was.

That day, I broke ties with her in a long, apologetic message left on her voicemail because I was too chicken to break it off face-to-face. I know, very Joe-Jonas-dumping-Taylor-Swift-via-text-message of me. I called my parents and hesitantly broke the news: I was only going to see Dr. Blatter from now on. Silence on the other end. I had to make my case. If I found myself struggling one bit, I promised, I would increase my sessions to a few extra times a week. I even pleaded a little. *Pause.* I could always go back to Dr. Attia; that door wasn't completely closed. I was just going to test the waters and see how I would do without her. *Silence.* Then finally, words. They weren't 100 percent on board. I could tell by the tone of their voices. But they agreed; I did have three and a half months with Dr. Attia under my belt. Also, I was an adult, so they didn't have the power over my decision the way they would if I were a child.

Look, real talk, from a now recovered mindset, leaving Dr. Attia's guidance was definitely not the smartest move I made in my recovery. Would I suggest that anyone in my shoes drop their eating disorder therapist? That would be a resounding *no way* or, better yet, *hell no!* I would absolutely suggest staying with your eating disorder therapist until he or she thinks you are ready to be on your own. But it was just my path to take, and I was lucky that, for me, it turned out okay.

Now the last step of Maudsley was, at least in my case, establishing a healthy adult identity. So ready or not, adult world, here I came, guns blazing!

In order to establish a healthy adult identity, I had to discover my likes and dislikes, and learn about myself in a healthy way. I basically needed to put my inner people-pleasing perfectionist to rest by saying *bye, Felicia* to that side of me—while giving a big, warm hello to healthy coping mechanisms, hobbies, and people I enjoyed. Not as easy as it may sound.

Finding an exercise that helped me cope with my anxiety, but didn't injure me, was hard. I was into running for a while, but not long after I started, I pulled my groin on the treadmill, which forced me to stop. That tenderness and discomfort on the inside of the thigh is painful. It was frustrating because, ever since I started recovering, I'd felt like I was constantly hurting myself—first the seizure, which took months to heal from, and now this. Then I discovered the perfect exercise.

Some people find God when they go through life-altering experiences; I found stationary cycling (sarcasm alert, but it was pretty mind-blowing for me). Spinning helped me conquer my stress without putting pressure on my groin. Each spin class, I would clear my mind with the music—blaring hits, oldies, obscure songs, or a mix—and I felt like I could rock out in my own private dance party on the bike. For forty-five minutes, I would get into the beat, sing to my badass self, and forget about everything. It was a chance to really breathe and decompress before going home for the night after a long day at the office. It was a healthy way of *really* clearing my mind.

"When exercising, focus on coordination, balance, breathing, strength and stamina, enjoyment, and improved health and body acceptance, rather than on calories burned or resulting changes in appearance," writes Carolyn Costin in *The Eating Disorders Sourcebook*. That was what I was trying to do. My main focus was on my mental health, which would translate to physical health and all-around health. It also gave me a semblance of a social life.

Instead of going straight home after work and being by myself (sorry, Ted, dog interaction didn't cut it), I would go spin the stress out. Bright red, sweat dripping from places I didn't know could sweat—a really interesting way to socialize, *right*? It would force me to be around other people and interact, which, I was told, is a part of being a normal functioning adult. The jury is still out on that.

Getting confident enough to potentially let someone into my life relationship-wise was another natural step into adulthood. As much as I hated to admit it—because it was something my dad used to say that made me cringe—I had to look my best to feel my best. This was just me starting to take care of myself by making "me" a priority—knowing my worth.

When my hair finally grew in an inch or so and was back to its usual thick texture, I got extensions to cover up the thin, unhealthy hair that had developed while I was sick. Most people wouldn't notice it, but I did, and I was doing it for myself. That's another part of adulthood, it turns out: doing stuff for you.

Hair was an easy physical change. Now, when I looked in the mirror, I shook out long, beautiful locks, instead of the short wisps I had been stuck with after making a rash decision to chop it all off years before—and then, because I was sick, it never grew back. What was interesting was that, now more than ever, I had control over every single aspect of my life, and I finally really believed and felt it—not just with my hair, but in my freedom to be whoever the hell I wanted. I was driving the car. My eating disorder was finally in the passenger seat.

FULL LIFE, AUGUST 2014

I sat down on my couch and sank deep into the cushions. Sometimes I felt like the couch called to me. "Dani, Dani, Dani, just sit and close your eyes for a second."

"Oy, Ted, what a day, what a day," I said to him, watching his little paws wildly going up and down, pawing at me to pick him up. "Okay, you little munchkin man, chill out." I grabbed him and put his little body next to mine.

"Dad drove me bananas today, and he's calling now. Ugh, I don't want to pick up." My landline was ringing, and Teddy barked wildly at the sound. "Hi, Dad, you just caused a lot of chaos with that one call. It better be worth it," I joked as I picked up the phone. "Oh, you are on your way home? Good. What are you and Mom going to do tonight? Sounds good. I am just going to work out, then relax and order in. Okay, have a good night. Love you...okay, okay, you too." I hung up the phone and placed it in its charger, taking a long, deep breath.

"Okay, little Ted nugget. I am going to go downstairs and work out for thirty minutes, and then I will come up and we can chill. Sound good to you?" I looked at Ted, staring at me blankly.

I changed into workout gear and was tying my shoelaces when: *ring-ring-ring.* "Oh, shit, you've got to be kidding!" I screamed, walking toward the phone. "I swear I am going to disconnect this thing!" I picked it up.

"Hello, yes, I will do it after I work out. I am about to leave the apartment. I will talk to you later. Okay, thanks." I hung up and finished tying my shoes.

"They don't give me a break, Ted. I am going to give myself one, though. Be back in a bit." I picked up my key fob, keys, and iPod and walked out the door before my landline or cell could ring again. I could keep on working, working, working, but sometimes you just need a little break and time for you. I recognized I needed "me time," so I took it. The next day, when I had a free moment at work, I posted on my Living a FULL Life Facebook page:

> *"If there is one consistent feature seen in all eating disorders that causes and perpetuates their existence, it is the need for control. Eating Disorder behaviors create the illusion of control. Giving up the behaviors feels like losing control and becoming powerless."*
> *—Carolyn Costin, The Eating Disorder Sourcebook*

> *It is important to feel like you are in charge of your own path. A numbing mechanism like an ED or an addiction can block out a problem temporarily but will eventually leave you feeling even more powerless than ever. Today, do something positive for YOU—run, Spin, do yoga, cook, read, write, change your hair the way you like it. Do something that puts you first, even for just thirty minutes. Self-care makes a difference You deserve it. Have a beautiFULL Monday.*

I felt so much better after my workout the previous night. My mind was clear and fresh. I got my work done, ordered in, and had a nice relaxing night. Those thirty minutes for myself made a huge difference, changing my entire mindset. It is so important to feed your soul with what makes you feel good. I wasn't doing that enough before.

The book *The Giving Tree* by Shel Silverstein often raises controversy over the question of whether the relationship between the tree and the boy should be interpreted as positive (the tree gives the boy selfless motherly love) or as negative (the boy takes advantage of the tree and the tree lets him destroy her). I look at it more positively, with the tree being like a mother figure to the boy, content just to make the boy happy. However, if it were not just the boy—if multiple people took, took, took from the tree, the tree would wind up with nothing, and maybe no one would care. The boy appreciated the tree as a stump, but others wouldn't.

I almost wound up being a stump because I gave too much of myself. Acknowledging my needs is just as important as acknowledging other people's needs. For the longest time, I did everything for everyone else (people-pleasing, volunteering, working), so much so that I often forgot about myself. I became a stump because there was nothing left of who I really was. I didn't even know what made me happy. I refuse to be a stump ever again.

As I mentioned earlier, one of the hardest parts about recovery was that I had nothing to come back to. I had been in an abusive relationship with myself on and off for twenty-two years, and permanently committed to self-destruction over the last four. It was hard to rebuild after twenty-six years of habitual self-hatred.

Since my attempts to connect with my school friends had been an epic failure, I still needed to find out who my adult friends would be. One thing was certain: I knew who they wouldn't be. A lot of my old friends had taken me for granted, and I let it happen because my self-esteem was low. Heck, I treated myself like shit, so why wouldn't everyone else?

I had a new attitude. I wasn't going to waste my time with negativity. The facilitator for a webinar I took through the National Eating Disorder Association summed it up perfectly: "Surround yourself with positive people. It is easier to feel good about yourself and your body when you are around others who are supportive and who recognize the importance of liking yourself just as you naturally are."

I finally felt I was deserving of these kinds of people because I was finally kind enough to myself to accept them. I didn't have anything to hide from them, no reason to push them away, now that I was in recovery. I was finally embracing my flaws, so I had to believe that other people would as well, and if they didn't, well...fuck 'em.

It had been a month since I'd seen Courtney, and we made plans for dinner. The last time, we'd had sushi, so she decided on Mexican this time around. (I wasn't quite there yet in my recovery, to choose such an adventurous cuisine.) I had never tried Mexican and didn't have a clue about what to order, which made me nervous. *But that's what this new, recovering Dani is about. She is in charge of her life, and she isn't going to let anorexia dictate who she is or where she goes.* I didn't even look up the menu online beforehand. *I was in charge, not anorexia.*

I hailed a taxi to take me downtown to a little Mexican restaurant on Avenue A in the East Village. Courtney was seated at a small table in the front corner. She got up to embrace me into a heartfelt hug. Her long blonde hair swept into my face, blinding me for a moment. We were seated next to the window, and I could see the frost sticking to the panes.

"How have you been? Sorry about it being so long again. I have to be a little better about keeping in touch," I said.

"Good, good, and me too. It's really okay," she answered and then looked down at her menu. I guessed that would be my cue to read mine too. *Crap,* I would have done anything to avoid this part—I knew it was going to be a challenge.

The more I read, the more I panicked. It was worse than I thought. Everything on the menu seemed to be filled with so many caloric and fatty foods: cheese, sour cream, avocado, rice. *Breathe, Dani, you will be okay, it's just food. It won't hurt you.*

"Do you want to get guacamole and chips to start?" Courtney asked sweetly, taking me out of the debate in my head.

Do I want to get guacamole and chips? Hell no! But was I going to go for it? "Sure," I answered. I had never had guacamole, and all I could think about was how filled with fat it was. *Avocados are healthy fats,* I reminded myself. Anything with the word *fat* in it made me cringe, but I had to be more open to these so-called good fats even though that sounded like an oxymoron to me.

The chips arrived, and I took one and hesitantly dipped it into the guacamole, my hand a little shaky, chip bouncing with it. It reminded me of the kids on Nickelodeon getting slimed by gooey green glob—fatty gooey green glob in this instance, ew gross—it was so easy for me to turn myself off of food. I could make anything look throw-up-inducing, but instead, I forced myself to take a bite. It tasted *way* better than it looked, and I surprisingly found myself with an ear-to-ear smile plastered on my face, and little remorse.

We continued talking between sips of wine, and I finally admitted to her what was going on, what the past few months had been like, and why I was really so out of touch. She deserved the truth. And I owed it to myself to let my walls of shame down and be vulnerable.

Also, I was sad—sad about what I had gone through and was still going through. I needed to let myself have a friend I could trust and be open with. I had been so caught up in my struggles and convinced I couldn't trust anyone that I'd lost any form of true connection. I needed to act as a friend to someone as much as I needed one—to equally care and reciprocate love and support. Sharing begets sharing, authenticity begets authenticity, and these are all positive rewards from letting yourself be vulnerable.

As I opened up, I started to cry, my heart dropping to the pit of my stomach. And then Courtney broke down in tears as well. She stood up and hugged me. She accepted me, shoulders welcoming my tears. I got out of her hug and wiped my eyes, breathing a sigh of relief.

"I knew all along," Courtney, said, wiping her big blue eyes. "I didn't know what to do. I wasn't sure if I should tell your parents, but I figured they were on top of you."

"No, you couldn't have done anything," I assured her. "I would have pushed you away. I did push you away, to some degree. I pushed everyone away." I paused. "Just being here for me now means so much."

I ordered a vegetable fajita. I didn't totally feel comfortable eating it, but I slowly nibbled around the fajita and ate the vegetables, then went back to the fajita again after conquering the much easier vegetable portion. I did all right overall. Despite the "scary" new foods, it was so good to see Courtney, and it was a fun dinner, although very different from the ones with my parents breathing down my neck, watching each bite. Outside of family, Courtney was the first person who knew about my "secret" from my own mouth. Telling her and receiving such warmth in return made me feel like it's okay to be flawed. Also, she had problems too! And she shared them with me. Lo and behold, I liked her even more for sharing them!

In that moment, I realized that no one is perfect, and that is actually the most beautiful and life-changing realization I've ever had. The people who have to pretend to be flawless are the ones I feel sorry for. I want to shake them and yell, "Snap out of it! It's okay to be imperfect! Your flaws set you apart in a great way. You will be so much happier once you embrace them!"

It took me far too long to believe this.

After that night, I did a lot of reading about eating disorders, trying to figure out what I went through, what exactly it was, how many people are afflicted, and so on. When I was struggling, I was too scared to confess even to myself that I had an issue, and investigating felt like an admission of guilt.

Through my research, I became aware that all the negative stigmas I believed about eating disorders were false. Most important, I learned that this is a medical illness—not something I caused myself. With that realization came forgiveness and an understanding of why I turned to my eating disorder. I have OCD, depression, anxiety, and low self-esteem and am a raging perfectionist who put so much pressure on myself to be everyone else's version of perfect instead of just being me. I couldn't cope with overwhelming emotions and stressful situations—and starving, bingeing, and purging helped ease my anxiety. All of this coupled with my genetic predisposition and our culture—I was bound to get an eating disorder.

I also started reading self-help books and became familiar with concepts like "shame" and "owning your story" and "being okay with being you." When shame sets in, it's our nature to want to shut it down. I numbed out to protect myself. Through anorexia, bulimia, and by being a workaholic, I did what Brené Brown calls "armoring up." I didn't leave any time to focus on what was really bothering me. What I knew for sure was that it was time for me to let go of all of that self-hate.

Shortly after my immersion into the written world of eating disorders, I decided to start my own Facebook page, Living a FULL Life (but you know this already; you've been reading excerpts from that page throughout this book). It was my way of fostering a relationship with people again. This was my way of saying I wanted to connect with the world by being a part of it and, at the same time, better it. It was my way of owning my story and of letting go of all the shame associated with my struggles by doing so. It was my way of moving forward, ridding myself of the stigmas surrounding eating disorders, so maybe others wouldn't have to go through what I did before they ask for help.

So that's what I sought out to FULLY do.

FULL LIFE, NOVEMBER 2013

We were going out for dinner at the Meatball Shop on the Upper East Side. I put on leggings and a long white sweater and threw my long hair into a bun. I painted eyeliner on my lower lid and dabbed on lipstick. I grabbed my keys and put them into my "recovery bag." My parents had gotten me a beautiful new purse midway through my recovery because they were proud of me for how far I had come. They said that nothing that would hurt me—laxatives being the emphasis—would be allowed to go into this bag. It was a starting-over bag. I loved that concept.

I gave myself a once-over in the mirror, kissed Ted on his furry forehead, and I was off. I walked the New York City streets, heading uptown. I loved how they looked at night, taxicabs zooming by and bright glaring lights. I felt like I was walking in a "Big Apple: Welcome to NY" postcard.

Was that my mom and dad outside the restaurant? Squinting to see them, I gave them a half-wave, and they waved back. As I approached, they reached for me, planting kisses on both of my cheeks.

The trendy restaurant wasn't as crowded as usual; some nights, there were lines out the door and into the street. I looked at the menu; it was one of those menus where you have to circle what you want. There were so many choices of meatballs: regular, chicken, vegetable, and pork, and then there were specialty meatballs listed on a chalkboard.

"Decisions, decisions," I said, my eyes on a "meatball smashed," which is kind of like a meatball hero. "I am deciding between veggie and pork. I know pork is kind of random, but it sounds good," I said, thinking aloud. I knew the veggie would be better, calorie-wise. I also knew it was safer in all regards, number one being that I had eaten it before.

"Well, whatever you are in the mood for. I am going to get a regular meatball smashed with tomato sauce and mozzarella," my mom said, circling her order.

Regular was code for beef in Meatball Shop terminology.

"Hmm...maybe I will do the same, but with pork," I said, thinking out loud again. "How about you, Dad?"

His eyes were fixed on the menu. He seemed a little confused by the ordering system. "A smashed, and then three meatballs naked on the side," he said, still looking over the menu. He had been growing his curly hair out lately. It was wild and free, like a little boy who'd just gotten off the swings or had gone running in the wind. I liked it.

"Okay, it is decided: I am going to try something new with the pork," I said, making the final circles and putting the menu on the table away, so I wouldn't change my mind.

The food was delicious. Pork, a little spicy, was a good move, and I was proud of myself for trying something different. A little spice goes a long way too—I knew now that I had found my inner sass. The next night, back at my apartment, I wrote a post on my Living a FULL Life Facebook page:

> What makes you a #RecoveryNinja? Be the strong ninja I know each of you are <3
>
> I am a #RecoveryNinja because I can now eat anything I crave. Last night a spicy pork meatball smash with mozzarella cheese from The Meatball Shop, and it was DELICIOUS, and I did not feel guilty at all, just satisfied. Tell me why you are a #RecoveryNinja and use the hashtag #RecoveryNinja #LivingAFULLLife. Happy Friday!

I posted it and closed my laptop. To think that, only a few months back, eating out in public would have caused me to shake. This feeling that things could only get better, if I kept putting my mind toward positive change, was a great feeling. I could do this. I was sure.

Not everyone was so understanding and accepting of my journey.

I went out for dinner with Elizabeth, who knew from my Facebook page and from her parents that I was in recovery from an eating disorder. I hadn't heard from her when I was recovering and living at home—not even a text to see how her "bestie," as she called me (for effect in front of her parents, I was starting to realize), was feeling. Her parents liked the idea that Elizabeth was best friends with a "good girl," so she'd kept up that farce and I, the perfectionist who so wanted everything to be okay that I'd fought any signs to the contrary, had remained accepting. But this, not hearing from her at all, when I was always there for her, hurt a lot. Plus, I was done making excuses on her behalf—I just fought for me, I had no energy left to fight for anyone not worth fighting for.

So, in the restaurant, now that I was *better*, she took it upon herself to ask a million trillion questions about my eating disorder. Eating out with a friend when you are recently in recovery is already stressful; the added anxiety of talking about my "issue" made it hard for me to chew, let alone swallow. Which brings me to something else: You don't have to tell anyone anything. It's your personal journey, and you don't owe it to anyone to say anything if you don't feel comfortable.

"So, Dani," Elizabeth said, as she took a sip of her second drink, "you seemed like the perfect kid, but really you were hurting yourself—just in less obvious ways than drinking and drugs?"

Her eyes, lined with bags, were bright red from weed. I used to like it that she didn't notice my eating, but, now that she did, I wondered if she was using my eating disorder to make herself feel better—like, *I got my shit so much more together than Dani; she's such a fuck-up.*

Yes, asshole, I was probably more fucked-up than you, but at least I don't ask stupid fucking questions, is what I wanted to say.

"I guess," I answered, while a new healthy inner voice whispered, *Do you really need friends like this?*

Answer: No.

It is interesting how the simplest stupid comment, after you have been through so much drama, can end an ongoing destructive relationship. It was time for me to say goodbye.

I never told Elizabeth what bothered me about her or our relationship. She didn't know how much she had hurt me throughout the years by our relationship being so one-sided. I would always care about her and be there for her, but I wasn't going to try so hard anymore, unless things drastically changed.

Maybe what kept us together was that I used to be her polar opposite, but now that I was a more balanced individual, it wasn't true anymore. I had a few of the qualities I had admired about her— her rebellious, not-giving-a shit-what-people-think attitude; her unconventional streak; and her uncanny sense of self—for myself now. I no longer needed Elizabeth to feel accepted or whole anymore.

When you have a mental illness, you get sucked into the belief that you don't belong. The truth is that you haven't let yourself find "your people" because you are convinced you are so different or deserve the shitty friends you keep around out of insecurity. I promise you, when you stop being so hard on yourself and stop these self-destructive beliefs and let people in, they will come. You will find them only if *you* want to be found, and you will form your own alien nation of weirdness together.

After that dinner with Elizabeth, I was finally ready to find my "own happy alien nation" and start letting *my people* into my life. You have to let in some bad to find the good. I was ready to find the good and hold on *really* tight.

CHAPTER 13

Touched Back to Life

Every human needs true connection and companionship, and I am no exception. Getting back into the dating game was my next step in finding a healthy adult identity.

After years of perfectionism keeping me isolated, I was ready to make mistakes and get a little messy. So I did what every other single twenty-something living in Manhattan does: I made a profile and joined the ranks of New York dating singles on JDate and Match. com.

I had major anxiety because I was convinced I was inexperienced, having slept with only one person. I imagined my opening spiel: *Hi, I am Dani, I am a recovering anorexic, I haven't dated anyone in four years, I work too much, and I am on a lot of medication to keep me sane. Oh, and I am most likely awful in bed and haven't had sex in over four years.* That was the truth, but thankfully, I refrained from writing it on my dating profiles.

I went on some interesting dates. There was the guy who told me I looked like his sixty-year-old history professor who he thought was the "perfect woman," and proceeded to show me a picture of her on his iPhone. For the record: I didn't really see the resemblance.

Then there was the guy who told me a rape story within our first five minutes. "I'm sorry," I replied politely, "but I really need to walk my dog."

"Can I come?" he asked, probably literally thought he was going to, too! *Gross.*

"No, sorry, but I will pay for my drink," I said throwing a twenty on the table, getting the hell out of Dodge as quickly as possible.

To be honest, I only considered going on that date with him because his profile picture looked like the actor who played Ron Weasley in the Harry Potter movies. Thought process at the moment (maybe two glasses of wine deep): *Oh, Rupert Grint lookalike! Ron Weasley must be a nice guy.* Wrong! Next time I would use different criteria for picking my dates.

Then there was the guy who critiqued my hair: "You know, your hair looks much better longer than that short look in your profile pictures." Um, thanks for your unsolicited opinion, asshole!

I began to learn about the types of men who would go on these dates: Some prompted me to wonder about their sexual preference; others still belonged in a college frat, playing beer pong with their frat brothers, fist bumping and saying "dude." Then there was a third category that consisted of men I could potentially be into.

The problem was, I wasn't open to meeting these other guys because I found it difficult to take any date situation seriously. And becoming an online dating success story is highly unlikely when you self-sabotage by finding something wrong with *everyone*. I felt like a caricature of myself on these outings. Part of my resistance might have been that, if I saw these meet-ups as more than a joke, I would have had to face being potentially rejected or, worse, let someone in and get my heart broken. In general, I just felt so damaged that I didn't think I could be a possible match for anyone. But there is someone for everyone, they say (who are *they* by the way, I always wondered—and how the hell do *they* know this stuff?).

The first guy I hit it off with was a former Israeli army commander whose family was in the diamond business. He had moved from Israel to New York two months prior to our meeting. Our first date took place at Tbar on the Upper East Side. I picked the location because it was close to where I lived. Also, if I had a completely miserable time, at least I knew I liked the ambience, and it always had some interesting characters for entertainment. I mean, last time I was there, so was an actual "Real Housewife"—Ramona Singer—and nothing is more entertaining than *Housewives* in their natural habitat.

For over an hour, I waited for him. I was pretty peeved, but I had two glasses of wine to pass the time. I considered leaving but decided against it. I preferred to people-watch rather than go back to my apartment, where I could be tempted to self-destruct. In the early stages of recovery, I tried to avoid alone time as much as possible.

I had a front-row seat to some quality people-watching anyway—couples on first dates, married couples, family dynamics. I would imagine what was happening by examining facial expressions, by lip-reading, and by overhearing snippets of conversations. It was like directing my own mini-films with characters who were even more interesting than the ones on television and in the movies. And when you are a *Real Housewives* junkie like me, that's saying *a lot*. And no, Ramona didn't make an appearance this visit.

After waiting *way* too long—according to the dating world's unwritten rulebook—I saw him. He looked like a leading man in a romantic feature. I pictured him walking in slow motion. Did I mention I'd been drinking? Everyone gets a little more attractive with wine goggles.

His name was Aaron. Aaron-the-Israeli-war-hero.

"I am so sorry. I don't know the subway system yet," he apologized, softly caressing my back. "And I came from Riverdale." He spoke with a thick Israeli accent as we locked eyes.

"I understand," I murmured, transfixed. "I find the subway system to be full of mysteries, like a maze or a never-ending fun house, and I've lived in New York way longer than you." *Come to me now, you tall, dark, handsome, dreamy person...*

His casual white T-shirt showed off his muscular torso and biceps. *Gosh, he could have tried a little harder for this date,* I thought, analyzing him from head to toe, trying to get a proper first impression. *Was that a ketchup stain on the top of his T-shirt? Yep. He definitely wasn't late because he took time to get ready, but hopefully those fries he ate were good.* I scanned him head-to-toe again. *On second thought, please don't let that ketchup stain be blood and him really a killer.* But did I mention how handsome he was? Killer or not (though I was hoping he was just a killer of French fries and chicken nuggets), after waiting all this time, I was going to give this date a real shot.

He sat down on a bar stool next to me and we got right to chitchatting. The rapport was instant. I liked his confidence—borderline arrogance, really—and there was something hot about how sure of himself he was. He told me impressive war stories. Part of me didn't believe him, because they seemed so obscene. The other part of me didn't give a shit because we were connecting! Suddenly I felt him grab my hand and my heart started pounding as my legs went weak. Before I could object or pull away, it started to feel nice, so I let him hold on to it. To be touched after so long, even a handhold, made my body shake with lust, fear, and nerves.

He continued talking about Israel, moving here, and his family, as I looked deeply into his eyes. *Those eyes...those beautiful, dark brown damaged eyes.* Was he more damaged than me from all those years at war? The thought comforted me. I knew and understood damaged people. I was one.

We both had another drink and then we headed out. I could feel the alcohol rush to my head as I stood up. I was drunker than I'd thought, and I found myself stumbling as I followed him out of the restaurant. The chilly New York streets jolted me upright, and a bit of my sobriety returned.

As we rounded the corner, he grabbed me around the waist and gave me a passionate kiss. Right there in the middle of East 73rd Street, we started making out, as he leaned me against a street lamp. It felt so nice to be kissed, to be felt, to have someone's arms around me.

I ended up spending the entire weekend with Aaron. We went to the Museum of Natural History, playing tourists. I liked to think of him as an alien, with me as his designated earthling, showing him around. *Maybe we can form our own alien nation of weirdness together?* He told me I was his "favorite person" in the States, and we laughed a lot and flirted with each other. That is, before he dropped a bomb: if I didn't sleep with him soon, we would have to settle for friendship and need to start seeing other people.

I should have responded, "It's your loss, buddy" and walked away or settled for friendship. We both needed friends—he'd just moved here, and I was rebuilding—we were both starting our lives. But no, I liked him, and I was vulnerable. I had no fantasies that we were going to be together forever—gosh, I wasn't even sure if I wanted that—but I decided I was going to sleep with him to get it over with. It's not like I didn't want to completely, too. I just didn't like how he went about it. Maybe new Dani didn't need to be in love to have sex. Maybe sex could be just that, sex. I was going to test this hypothesis.

I didn't like the pressure he put on me, but I figured it must be weird for a woman in her late twenties to be holding out. If he was going to use me for sex, I would use him for it back, as a science experiment. I was always good at assignments, so this should be a breeze. Old Dani couldn't do that because she was too much in her head. New Dani—a badass, comfortable with her sexuality—*totally* could... Right?

I started imagining this new version of myself. I would let loose. Enjoy the moment like those sexually powerful femme fatales. I was in my late twenties in Manhattan. I would become sexually experienced, like Carrie Bradshaw. Oh, so *Sex and the City* chic. I would be the girl that hit on guys at the bar whenever she felt like it. I would be the girl that took guys back to her apartment and had her way with them. Dani Sherman, the man-eater. *Yeah, right!*

Two nights later, in preparation, I drank two glasses of wine, pretending it was fancy champagne just to feign romance, and tipsily texted Aaron to come over. *It'll be like ripping a Band-Aid off.* About half an hour—and a half glass of wine later—he showed up at my door. He kissed me on my lips, picked me up, and threw me on the bed.

He was there to have sex with me, nothing else, and that's what we did. And it was terrible for me. I felt like he didn't respect me, it hurt, and I spent the entire experience second-guessing myself. He left not long after, and I was left alone, sitting on my bed, still a little drunk, with so much shame—and a bad taste in my mouth. I quickly pulled the plug on Aaron after that encounter. Conclusion to my hypothesis: New Dani was no Carrie Bradshaw, and casual sex wasn't for her. She'd always be doomed to be more of a prim and proper Charlotte York. Hell, maybe that wasn't a bad thing, though. That didn't make me any less of a badass, I finally realized. It was just who I was. And being who you are, and owning it completely in this crazy world, is the bravest thing you can do.

I cried the whole next day. I felt like I shouldn't have gone through with it just because he was putting pressure on me. And now he was texting me and I didn't want to be with him in any capacity. I hated that he put pressure on me. I hated that I did it. I was so mad at myself for doing something that I wasn't completely sure about. Also, I was swollen, fat, and alone.

"Fat is not a feeling," I kept repeating. *"Fat is your default. But if you tune in, you'll realize that you're actually anxious about your gynecologist appointment tomorrow—the one where you may feel out of control and maybe out of place. Oh, and now you have to mention that you're a slut because you are convinced you were given some sort of nasty STD."* See, way too much in my head for casual sex.

It was hard for me to believe this mantra about the gynecologist appointment, so I wrote it down to make it real. Freaking out over an STD was pretty paranoid, considering we had used protection (though, kids, it's smart to get your partner tested and know their sexual history before engaging in intercourse of any kind, so you know your risks). I was just driving myself nuts and self-destructing—an old pattern when I was nervous about something I didn't want to face.

But what I was most worried about was that the doctor would tell me I'd messed up my body irreversibly from all the years of abuse. I wanted a baby more than anything one day, and if I couldn't have one, was there really a point to all of this? Of course, there was! I just needed to get there and fighting for my future babies was an easier concept for me to stick to because my self-esteem was still so low. Fighting for myself, along, at this juncture was not always the best motivator. I had so many contradicting and crazy thoughts zipping through my head, all I could do was lie in bed and cry. So that's what I did for the rest of the day.

I pressed the buzzer on the ornate, gold-framed doors of number 993, a red-brick building topped by a green-cascaded roof that harkened to Roaring Twenties Park Avenue—carefree times when women empowered themselves with music, fashion, culture, independence, and the right to vote.

"Fancy," I said with a shimmy, channeling my inner 1920s flapper girl. I needed all the empowerment I could get on a day like today.

A strong buzz sounded through the intercom, and I opened the door to be greeted by a woman with electric red hair and pale skin, sitting at what I assumed was her desk.

"Hi, I'm Danielle," I said to the woman, who resembled Kathy Griffin, a scent of French vanilla perfume wafting from her wrists.

"I have an appointment with Dr. Chang. I really like your perfume, by the way." I twisted my curly brown hair to the side of my face.

"The doctor will be with you shortly," she answered robotically. "Just have a seat in the waiting room." Then, to my delight, she offered a slight smile.

The waiting room was filled with women boasting baby bumps in all shapes and sizes. I seated myself next to a small brown wooden table piled with stacks of magazines, a good vantage point to unobtrusively stare at the other patients. One dirty-blond woman in particular caught my eye. She was with her male partner, their hands tightly clasped, looking so happy.

My eyes scanned my own body. Pregnant ladies in Dr. Chang's waiting room, one point; sad-lonely-fucked-up-recovering-anorexic Dani, zero. Zero because I didn't have a bump or a partner and wasn't sure if I would *ever* have either, especially after my awful fling with Aaron that had left me extremely insecure. Tears welled with the word *ever*. I hoped no one would notice. I grabbed the magazine on top of the stack and pretended to browse it. *Great! Parenting. Why doesn't the world just throw my fear of being infertile in my face?*

"Danielle, follow me, please," announced an assertive voice, forcing me to suck up my tears.

Dr. Chang had straight black hair and was dressed to the nines in high Louboutin shoes and a black pencil skirt, masked only by her lab coat, which she wore just as elegantly. *How does she not twist her ankle?* I pictured myself awkwardly wobbling in heels in front of the mirror, until ending up ass-slammed on my bedroom floor and surrendering them back to the closet where they belonged. I couldn't help but feel unworthy. Dr. Chang, five points for being so absolutely freakin' perfect; Dani, still zero.

She made her way over to her desk and sat down, looking at my records on her computer, silent for a couple of minutes. "Danielle, you haven't been here in five years."

I nodded.

Her eyes darted from her computer, to me, and then back in disappointment.

"I had anorexia." The sentence spilled out like the vomit I not long ago induced in myself through incessant laxative abuse. "I am in recovery now, but I am so scared I messed up my body. I want a baby one day, and if I can't..."

Dr. Chang stood, took a couple of steps toward me, and put her cold hand on my bare shoulder, which made me whimper a bit harder. "We will figure this out. The future will be," she paused, trying to think of a comforting word, "um...better."

Not convincing, but I nodded in response to her effort, wishing I had honored my body more and that I hadn't wanted to die *so* badly that I would now find myself potentially unable to conceive my own children. Conclusion, or final score card: Dani is a complete zero.

Hold up, no more self-loathing. Enough with the pity party, Dani. You are doing better and your life scorecard is just beginning, a voice suddenly piped up. I imagined a devil and an angel on each shoulder. A devil, because Mom called anorexia "the devil inside of me." I needed to choose the angel—the voice I was finally hearing— which was a rational and positive voice. *There is no need to compare yourself to others. That is ED speaking, and I thought we were working on ignoring that?* I nodded my head in agreement with this line of thinking. *And just because she is dressed well doesn't mean she is perfect. You of all people should know that—you don't even really know her. No one is perfect. Also, you love other people's imperfections, when are you going to start to really love your own?* I desperately needed this self-pep talk. I had to recognize that, as much as it was still hard in tough situations like this to ignore the negative ED voice that still taunted me, I'd have to fight it and not let it bring me down. What was significant in this moment was that I was beginning to see I *could* counter ED's lunacy with rational thinking—choosing the halo over the pitchfork.

Dr. Chang then led me to the exam room and told me to undress, except for a white sheet around my waist. I did what I was told and sat there, feet in stirrups, ready to be examined.

A few moments later, Dr. Chang knocked on the door and walked in. She gave me a full body exam. My body check and pelvic exams were normal; I could one day have babies, if I remained at a healthy weight.

I am okay. I was so relieved I started to cry again, this time happy tears.

With the same sad and sorry facial expression Dr. Chang had had at the beginning of our appointment, she put her hand on my shoulder, tapping it awkwardly. "You see? Things can only get better." What a *great* bedside manner, huh?

Yet this time, I nodded, believing it could.

Right away, I called my mom and told her the good news: I didn't screw up my body. Anorexia didn't take everything from me. Yes, it stole experiences and time in my past, but my future now had endless possibilities, and babies fell into that—because anything I wanted did. It made me feel, for the first time, that I had a chance. I had to start making better decisions. Bye, Aarons of the world. New Dani has a future and she's going to start *really* learning to love herself by giving her body and soul the respect they deserve. Because I'd want my future babies to do the same.

That week, during work, I decided I wanted to do something to solidify the idea that I was going to be okay, would respect my body, and wasn't going to hurt myself again. I had been thinking about this for a while, though I had never verbalized it. I was going to get a tattoo of the NEDA symbol near my lower left hip, so that when I looked in the mirror and saw what I thought were flaws, I would embrace them. The tattoo would serve as a reminder of how far I had come and where I wanted to remain—in recovery. Also, I couldn't be a hypocrite with this symbol engraved on my body. Okay, truth be told, I totally could, but I wouldn't. Not like when young boys get their first girlfriend's name tattooed on their chest. This was more serious, like a marriage (without divorce as an option), and me and recovery would be married till death do us part.

My tattoo artist was bald, with dark skin and tattoos on every inch of his body. He mentioned he was from Brazil, as he sketched the mock-up design of the NEDA symbol: the half-heart symbolizing loving concern for those suffering from eating disorders, and the female body representing diversity and acceptance of all body shapes and sizes. With two thumbs up and a smile, I gave my seal of approval of the design that would be forever etched on my skin. He then told me to lie down, patting his hands on the long black table beside him. I hopped on and made myself as comfortable as possible, and he started the tattoo.

"I have never seen this design before. What does it mean?" he asked, eyes focused on his artwork.

"It means I am in recovery from an eating disorder," I said, looking down at the outline on my skin as his tattoo gun kneaded into it, causing a slight burning sensation.

"That's really cool," he said without hesitation, and continued to drill.

"Thanks." It *was* cool, and I felt a strong pride in my recovery.

After he was done, he had me look in the mirror. The mirror—an object I had loathed for so long. I looked hard at my reflection, and for the first time and to my amazement, I saw something beautiful on my body in dark black ink. I was pleased and smiled at the person staring back at me.

FULL LIFE, MAY 2013

I had signed up for the advanced soccer league on ZogSports. I was giving the program another whirl since the first time I'd played with Courtney. Now I was in a new and different place, a better place. A place of moderation. Doing anything halfway, to me, used to mean a "failure." I was learning that it is actually called moderation, or the middle ground people call the "gray area." It is more than okay and is actually the healthiest option. I was working on doing things for fun. I just needed to find things I considered fun.

I was a little nervous because, after eight years, I was rusty. Also, I was not in the best shape. I just was getting myself strong after being sick for quite some time. I'd bought a soccer ball and had been practicing my moves around the apartment.

The gym was around the corner from where I lived. I wore my shin guards and indoor soccer shoes—more hardcore than the others, who wore sneakers sans any kind of guard (but I told you, I was still a work in progress on the whole moderation concept). They all seemed to know each other from prior seasons.

A little while and some introductions later, I was passing the ball around with a guy, chatting. Then, before I knew it, the Zog ref blew the whistle and the game started. I volunteered to be a substitute, preferring the sidelines to observe the level of play. That's when I realized my team was very good! We scored within the first five minutes. I was afraid to play.

"Dani, you're in," yelled a teammate.

I paused, out of fear, then ran onto the indoor field. And a second later, someone passed me the ball. I couldn't get rid of it fast enough. This indoor soccer league was all about speed and not as much skill. It was intense! I was struggling with that, as I wasn't in great shape yet, and my team was ridiculously competitive. Sweat dripping down my face and back, I glanced at a mirror. I was as red as a cherry lollipop, and this wasn't very fun at all.

After that game, I went home and showered, bypassing the drinking scene. Who was I kidding? That was never really what I was about. I rested my feet, walked Teddy, and ordered in Chinese. Then I wrote a post on the Living a FULL life Facebook page:

> *Here is a little advice for people newly in recovery from an eating disorder: I found it helpful to be very busy—keeping my mind occupied was basically the equivalent of sanity vs. self-destruction. I didn't want a moment on my own where I could think back and get sad which could ultimately lead to a binge, followed by a strong laxative temptation. It is ironic, for someone who preferred isolation and liked being on my own for so long, that the thought of being alone had become frightening. It was easy to keep busy on weekdays between work and dinner with my parents, or exercise at night, but the weekend presented a challenge. How would I kill time when I was still searching for friends and gaining my life back? Here is what a typical day looked like for me on a weekend:*
>
> *Sunday*
> *Volunteer at a homeless shelter: 10 a.m.–1:15 p.m.*
>
> *Lunch at Subway by myself: 1:30 p.m.–2:00 p.m. (Yes, I was proud I ate in public by myself too. A huge step.)*
>
> *Blow out: 2:30 p.m.–3:30 p.m. (I was starting to take care of myself.)*
>
> *Zog soccer: 4:30 p.m.–6:00 p.m.*
>
> *Work at home: 6:30 p.m.–8:30 p.m.*
>
> *Dinner: 8:30 p.m.–9:00 p.m.*
>
> *Write in journal: 9:00 p.m.–10:00 p.m.*
>
> *Get in bed and watch a movie.*
>
> *I didn't really like Zog soccer and quit after the first game, but you have to try new things to learn what is for you and what isn't. Either way, it was good to keep myself busy and to not give myself a moment to dwell on what I just went through, because that is very depressing. Those were the times when I would cry and think I didn't have a chance, when I really did. I promise, the voices dissipate weekly. It is not an easy process; it was the hardest thing*

*I ever did and requires patience (which I lack) and strength (which I have discovered I have a lot of). But if I can do it, you can beat the disordered cycle too. Once you are out of it, life gets so much better. Have a busy*FULL *recovery*FULL *beauti*FULL *night.*

Yes, I had a busy day, and I was tired. Right now, keeping myself busy was important, though. I just had to find what I liked to keep busy with, and I was working on it. I was constantly working on it all.

After my initial phase of recovery, I went through a little bit of a defiant phase, which was really me having a full-on identity crisis and using alcohol as a crutch to get me through it. When a couple divorces, the individuals often try on radical personas, testing out new versions of themselves. I had to find me without anorexia. We'd had a messy divorce and all I got out of it was my identity, and I wasn't sure what it was exactly. Who was I without my eating disorder? I had such a long history of people-pleasing that I had forgotten who I was. I'd developed chameleon skills, changing colors at the drop of a hat as a situation demanded. I hadn't even met adult, post-eating-disorder Dani—and I really wanted to. To do this, I needed to face situations I'd never let myself experience without anorexia.

So I let the experiences come, even ones that I hadn't liked in the past. I went drinking with my old friends from high school just to get out, and if a guy was talking to me and was an asshole, I would just dance instead of putting up with his bullshit "come-ons," especially if he came off as a player type. I had one guy ask if I wanted more drugs. I wasn't on any! I made my own fun. I didn't care anymore; I felt so out of place everywhere, why pretend I belonged?

I waved my freak flag extra high for shock value. I became a partier, drinking my emotions away, not giving a shit. Because why not? Playing by the rules didn't get me anywhere. This partying wasn't my scene, and the only way I felt comfortable was "another vodka on the rocks, please." And I found myself headfirst in the toilet by the end of the night. *Which is great! There goes your dinner and all the empty alcohol calories.* Shut up, ED! Being completely reckless got old very quickly.

Who was I without obsessing about food? I was still finding this key component of myself.

On the cab ride home from my last night out in this short-lived party-girl phase, I thought about being on a plane and traveling the world, just getting away. The fluffy clouds would morph into different shapes and sizes as I soared above them into the clear blue sky.

When I was little, I used to believe that Care Bears inhabited the clouds, and I would try to spot them outside the window of the plane. My mom would say that the turbulence was caused by the Care Bears fighting. Unfortunately, adulthood bestows on us the ugly truth: there are no Care Bears. Life is hard and turbulence is just that—turbulence. Getting on a plane and running away would not be my answer. I'd have to keep exploring within my own environment. Just being myself, volunteering, doing what I liked. It would all come together if I remained true to myself.

When I got home that night, I went right for Teddy. I always felt I belonged with him in our apartment. "Hi, my little man," I said, holding his furry little body high like Rafiki did to Simba in *The Lion King*. "It's good to be back in our kingdom, Ted." I gave him a kiss and put him back on the floor, then looked up again, smiling at the walls of my apartment. "Yes, it's good to be back." I was going to find me by doing what came naturally—being myself...

CHAPTER 14

When Pigs Fly

FULL LIFE, DECEMBER 2014

It was almost the New Year—2015. Where had time flown? I had my confetti and blow horns ready. It was freezing cold outside. Out the windows of my apartment, I saw people slip-sliding on ice, wearing heavy jackets, little girls and boys in mittens holding their parents' hands. I looked back at my laptop.

Sigh, blank screen again. I wanted to write a Facebook post for New Year's, but who was going to give a crap? *Risk: people thinking I sound like an idiot. Reward: really helping someone.* Good outweighed bad, so I began to type.

I have never believed in New Year's resolutions because I think you should better yourself every day. A part of me now doesn't like them even more because they are provoked by a number. On January 1st, you are supposed to start whatever your goal is and pursue it hard—weighing it on a figurative scale of your success every day. As with an eating disorder, you may be setting yourself up for disaster. This is why I advise you to evolve healthily each and every day of the year. In the New Year, respect your body, always be true to yourself, don't waste your time people-pleasing, and spend time with the people who love you wholeheartedly. Most importantly, know that you will never be everyone's perfect person, so just be YOU.

"What are you doing?" Sebastian interrupted my train of thought. "So focused on your day off," he continued, putting his head on top of mine and reading what I'd posted.

"I know, I know. Just finishing up a post for Living a FULL Life for the New Year," I said, embracing him in a backward hug. His thick black hair was combed with gel and he had on black sweatpants with a gray hoodie. Black socks covered his feet, keeping them warm because it was cold in my apartment; the floor tiles were numbing my own bare feet. He kissed the top of my forehead.

"Thank you," I said, smiling up at his dimpled cheeks and cleft chin.

"For what?"

"For that kiss," I said.

I heard the wind blowing against the floor-to-ceiling windows that framed the perimeter of my apartment. I closed my laptop and took his hand, leading him to the bedroom.

"What happens now?" he cheekily asked, following my lead.

"We get warm."

Not long after my defiant phase, when my heart was wide open and my mind was in a much better place, I met the love of my life, Sebastian. He is not my cure-all, by any means, and I am not saying that a ring and a wedding cured my eating disorder or made me well, because they didn't. What I am saying is that because I was happy and healthy enough, mentally and physically, to let myself be vulnerable, the conditions for true connection were set.

We had met at a Taxicab & Limousine Convention in March 2009. Yes, take that in and have a good laugh. It was my first official year in the business. It was also my first official year into my four-year spiral with adult anorexia. This convention would be my first public appearance as vice president of our company, and I desperately wanted to look "important." This was a lot of firsts, and nothing is more important to a perfectionist than a first impression.

I walked into the ladies' room of the convention center and stared at myself in the mirror. *My face looked round. Was my hair too flat?* I tried puffing it out with my hands to make it look thicker. I took a deep breath and applied more lipstick. I usually avoided mirrors in public bathrooms; I hated when people would stop in front of them, posing to analyze their faces and bodies. *So vain,* I thought. Maybe I was just jealous of their confidence. *Definitely.*

Exhaling, I stared at my reflection. *Here we go, Dani. Fake it till you make it.* I left the bathroom and headed to the main room alone. My mom was going to meet us at the after-party at Madame Tussaud's, and my dad was already in the main room, socializing and making his rounds.

I walked up the stairs in the Grand Hyatt and toward the stairs to the main room where all the booths were set up. I made sure I was standing up straight, not slouching like the hunchback of Notre Dame I normally was. *Quasimodo,* taunted the voice in my head, making me stand even straighter. As I walked in, I looked around for someone I knew—anyone! Someone to put my nerves at ease. I saw Charlie, a man I knew well from work, and approached him.

"You two should meet," Charlie commanded in his best networking voice, turning to the dark-haired man, wearing a black suit with a contrasting sharp red tie, standing next to him. "This guy does the same work as you, Dani, but out in San Francisco. You're both young and in the same business. Maybe you will hit it off." And he walked away wearing a shit-eating grin. *That fucker.* I tried not to stare too hard at the well-dressed man, who accentuated his dark skin and big baby browns with a stylish, well-maintained goatee.

"I'm Sebastian," he said, politely offering his hand.

We started talking about business and life in general. I'd just gotten over Blake and wasn't in a place to start anything with anybody, especially with someone across the country. *Nobody would like me for me; I don't even like me.* I politely ended our small talk, saying goodbye to Sebastian without a second thought—unless it was how to avoid going out to eat later with our colleagues and business associates.

Later, I survived the ordeal at the wax museum, thanks to my mother's company combined with the smoothness of Grey Goose. I pretended not to notice locking eyes with Sebastian across the room, but as he made his way toward me, I knew I couldn't avoid him.

I was bad at getting away from people; I never wanted to hurt anyone's feelings. *Imagine if someone did that to me. Straight to bingeing, followed by laxatives.*

Sebastian blatantly tried too hard to seem cool with insecure bragging,

"My limo driver got out of the car tonight to open the door for me, and I noticed he was wearing socks with sandals. It was so unprofessional."

"Oh," was my response, because I thought, *so what.* Clearly, he wanted me to know he'd arrived in a limo too. *Gross.* I'd later find out he owned a limo company that he'd started when he was sixteen, so that's why it bothered him. I forgot I was at a Taxi & Limousine Convention, limo being the operative word. My bad. I was also looking really hard for something not to like about him as protection, of course—so once he said that, I was relieved. *Phew, he's an asshole anyway, so I can't like him, and if I can't like him, he can't hurt me.*

In response, I acted more like myself, because I didn't care what he thought about me. But, although I wasn't having a completely terrible time, I decided it was time for me to split. *Peace out, Sebastian.*

I looked away from him, searching for an outlet. Ahead of me, I saw my mom and Sara, an associate, staring and smiling, obviously spying on our interaction. I smiled back, looking at Sara. I sparked a plan.

"I want to introduce you to someone," I said to Sebastian. "Be right back."

I then approached them, rolling my eyes. They giggled. My mom shot me a look like *Jeez, Dani, can't you give anyone a chance?* I shot her a look that could kill: *No, Mom, I can't. Leave me alone!* I turned to see Sebastian sipping his cocktail, eyes focused on me.

Craftily grabbing Sara, I dragged her over to him, introduced them, then left the two of them to talk. I had no room in my life for a man, a long-distance relationship, or anyone else who could potentially hurt me. *Nice move, Dani,* I told myself. And went back to my apartment to fall asleep with my vodka-and-Xanax cocktail.

Six months into my recovery, I received an email from Sebastian. It had been four years since I'd pawned him off on Sara, and I hadn't heard from him or run into him at any other business functions. I was, ironically, riding in a cab, resistance low after having a less-than-stellar evening out with my childhood friend, Alexis, and her medical-school clique—think *Grey's Anatomy* with a sloshed and obnoxious cast.

Safe in a taxicab, I entertained my mind by checking my emails, scrolling down on my phone until one caught my eye:

SUBJECT: Taxicab, Limousine, Paratransit, Association (TLPA) 2009—Grand Hyatt Meeting.

I didn't remember what he looked like, but I remembered I'd liked what I had seen very much—so much, I didn't want to face it. I opened the message and read:

Hi Danielle,

I'm not sure if you remember me, but I met you a few years back at the Grand Hyatt in Manhattan during TLPA's Spring Convention in 2009. I'm sorry if I'm intruding but I asked for your email address from someone we had in common. I just wanted to reach out to you because I never got a chance to say goodbye or to say how nice it was to meet you, especially someone in the same industry as I am in. I had tried to look you up a few times after the event to reestablish a connection, but I never was able to find any information online.

Anyways, I just wanted to reach out to you and say hello and to

---

see how you're doing. I'm sure you're busy learning the business everyday like I am and thought maybe you and I could talk sometime.

Looking forward to hearing back from you soon....

Take Care,
Sebastian

I like to joke that he had me at goodbye. I remember the first time we spoke on the phone. Actually, I don't. He called at eleven eastern and eight Pacific, since he still lived in California. I had taken some sleeping medication and answered the phone excitedly. And then, like out of a bad movie, everything went black. I woke in the middle of the night and flipped out, hitting myself on the head and dying a little inside. *Did we talk? Oh, no, fuck my life! Why do I have to constantly ruin everything?*

I texted him and got no response. I thought I must have scared him away, and who could blame the poor guy? I was mortified. I finally got a text back, telling me to call him in a couple of hours when he woke up. I was relieved. Even if we weren't going to be an item, for business reasons, I didn't want him to think I was a total freak.

"Hi, Sebastian, I am so sorry about last night," I explained when I called him back at a decent hour. "I took sleeping meds and I don't remember anything." I paused and then cringed—not the best conversation starter.

"You don't remember anything?"

The confused tone of his voice tempted me to take it all back as a sick joke, but verbal diarrhea prevailed: "No, I blacked out the second I picked up the phone. I am so humiliated."

Silence.

Shit.

"So, Sebastian, did we talk for a long time?"

"Like forty-five minutes."

I covered my face with my hands. *What the hell had we talked about?* I asked, thoughts aligning with my mouth, and he answered. And then I wanted to crawl under a giant rock and hide forever. *This is precisely why people shouldn't do drugs—even prescription ones! I was a walking ad campaign for D.A.R.E. (Drug Abuse Resistance Education).*

Apparently, Sebastian had asked me to tell him something nobody knew about me, and I happily obliged in my non-lucid state, sharing that I had a tattoo, and that led me to telling him "my secret." The only way to remain calm was to consider this whole mess a blessing. My "secret" would have to be shared sooner or later if I were ever to get into an intimate relationship, so maybe the fact that it was out now, and I couldn't take it back, was a blessing in disguise. At that point, I wore my tattoo like a warning sign: "I am in recovery from an eating disorder, stay away." Sebastian didn't see it that way.

"I feel bad, Dani," Sebastian told me in that voice that sent shivers down my back and made the butterflies do an extra lap around my stomach. "I know a secret about you, so I'll have to even out the playing field."

I felt a spark that I had never felt with anyone before. He told me about himself, and from then on, we talked every day—marathon calls that graduated to FaceTime, until the inevitable happened and he flew to New York to take me on a date.

It was the longest date I had ever planned. Since he was coming across country, we decided he would stay for a long weekend. Even though we had spent countless hours getting to know each other on FaceTime, my nerves were in overdrive. What if we didn't have real-time chemistry?

At 8:15 p.m., he rang the doorbell and I ran to get it, trailed by Ted barking like the huge dog he believed himself to be. I swung the door open, and there he was: white T-shirt, black vest, and dark jeans, holding a bouquet of white roses. Like a true gentleman, he kissed me on the cheek. I, on the other hand, tossed the flowers and went right for his mouth. You see, maybe I did have an inner Carrie Bradshaw. I was just waiting for someone I *really* liked and saw a potential future with to bring her out. We made out as he carried me to the living room. He plopped down on the couch with me on top of him.

"I can't believe I am actually with you," he said, holding me.

I couldn't believe I was with him either, and I grinned.

It was an amazing weekend. We went out for nice dinners, danced (yes, this former goody-two-shoes hit the club), and really got to know each other in all possible ways. I felt a level of happiness I had never known—laughing, smiling, holding hands, eating, kissing—enjoying every moment. Finally, *really* living, experiencing, and making memories. Not standing on the sidelines, watching other people's love stories play out, but creating my own. By the weekend's end, I felt like I'd known him forever. I was *so* sure I had found my partner to form my own alien nation of weirdness with.

Accompanying him back to the airport, I felt sad. I didn't want him to leave. Before he turned the corner to go through security, Sebastian said goodbye for the umpteenth time, and I watched him go. He then surprised me, turning one last time, for that last look I was waiting for, and said, "I love you."

Four months later, Sebastian proposed. He moved to New York that winter.

Teddy wasn't as fond of Sebastian as I was, to say the least. He would pee on Sebastian's side of the bed and growl at him while guarding me. Think: the three of us on the couch watching a movie, I'm in Sebastian's spoon, Teddy lying on me. I fall asleep, and Ted turns around and looks at him, "Grrrrrr." He was a real alpha, claiming his woman: me. Sebastian thought it was funny and found himself sucking up to a tiny dog, who would unfortunately take a *long* time to accept him.

In October 2013, I came home one night after work to find Teddy tripping repetitively, falling over his little feet like he had broken into my liquor cabinet and had gotten himself wasted. I rushed him to the animal hospital, thinking he'd hurt his legs somehow during the day. It wasn't his legs and sadly the diagnosis was much worse than too much liquor. The next day, the neurologist told me that he had a cyst in his brain, inflammation, and a separate autoimmune problem. The good part was that there was a temporary "fix." He was given pills that kept him steady. He would never be the same, though.

Ten months later, he had another setback. He'd had a seizure. We awakened from a loud yip. When I held him in my arms, he felt lighter, almost lifeless, like his soul was already gone. I was right. He didn't rebound well like I'd done from my seizure, and over the course of the day, he made no improvements.

"I'm so sorry. He isn't going to make it back from this," said the doctor, who my mom and I nicknamed Dr. Handsome because he resembled an edgy rock star. Think Adam Levine as a vet—tall, tatted, muscular, with dark hair. Even coming from him, Mr. Easy-on-the-eyes-so-everything-sounds-good handsome vet, the news was devastating.

My heart split as I nose-dived into Sebastian's chest to blockade my tears. I cried so hard that my puffy eyes felt like they were going to fall out by the day's end. I cried because I was losing my best friend. I cried because we had been through so much together, and now I was losing him. I cried because sometimes life was not fair, and this was that confirmation. I just cried.

I lost him a week before our wedding. People would tell me it was as if he knew I would be okay and had someone else to take care

169

of me. I didn't agree. I didn't need someone else to take care of me anymore—I was finally strong enough on my own. I just wished we were well together. I was sick and, right after I got better, he became ill. Maybe we were meant to take care of each other.

Life quickly went on. I stayed strong and remained in recovery, despite the emotional pain of losing Teddy and the empty feeling that followed of something missing, calling to *fill it, fill it, one last time.* I was going to fill it with other things besides binge food. I was going to have FULL relationships, embrace my imperfections, and follow my passions without thinking twice about other people's opinions. That's the way I would add fuel to my empty feeling. I knew for certain I could do anything if I remained in recovery.

I had always said I would get married when pigs fly. A lot of it had to do with me feeling like I'd always be sick and have *my secret* to hide. I was too broken for anyone to love me. Now that I was in recovery, I realized how wrong I had been. I am not broken. I am a beautiFULL bent mess like everyone else. We all have our struggles, our rough edges, but once we overcome them, we become stronger and better people. I am proud of the person I have become. On October 25, 2014, Sebastian wore flying pig cuff links on our wedding day. Also, I swear I saw a pig soaring that night, its little wings fluttering over Central Park. My best friend had become my husband, and we were making a life in my favorite city—a FULL life.

FULL LIFE, OCTOBER 25, 2014

"I can't believe my baby is getting married," my mom said as she draped her favorite necklace around my neck. The diamonds were from her mom's engagement ring, making it a very special necklace. Mom was smiling wide, her white teeth brightly contrasting with her dark red lips, rollers in her hair.

It was time for me to put on my wedding dress. My future mother-in-law and sister-in-law and my mom were all there to help me into it and take photos in the process. It all seemed so elaborate to me, but I went along with it. My mother and father had been through so much. They deserved to see me get married, give me away, whatever terminology you want to use. My dress was thrown over my head and squeezed onto my body.

It was an off-white, trumpet-cut, strapless gown we found at Kleinfeld Bridals. It was the first place we went to look for dresses and only the third one I tried on. My mom wanted me to keep looking, but I knew this was the dress, and I was done, tired, and over it from two hours of speed-shopping.

Shopping was not my thing. Everything about a wedding, all the "look at me, look at me" attention on the bride, was antithetical to my personality. Like I told my husband, I was so excited to marry him and be his wife, but I could do without the wedding thing. My parents were big wedding people, and that, coupled with the reality that for so long they hadn't known if their baby would live, let alone let herself get married and be happy, made me want to let them bask in the wedding and in the ceremony of "giving" me away.

Recently my mother wrote a guest post for my Living a FULL Life Facebook page that put words to the ordeal any parent goes through with a child who is suffering from an eating disorder:

> Watching your child battle with anorexia is like watching David trying to take down Goliath. The enemy is huge and scary and deadly. When that child is willing to help themselves while you work to save their life, the feat is attainable. Not to say this is, by any means, a day in the park. It is a process that takes strength and perseverance from everyone involved. Parents need to remember that there is a light at the end of the tunnel, and when you see your child return to health, there is nothing more beautiful or gratifying in your life. So, my words of wisdom are: never give up, EVER. Even on the days when you cry yourself to sleep. It's all worth it!! Let your child know you are there! Come hell or high water. You will get them through this. Dani, I have never been more proud of you. I know with every fiber of my being that if that beast tries to rear its awful head again, your strength will cut it down. You are truly my hero.
>
> I love you, Mom #NEDAwareness

You are my hero, Mom. I wouldn't be here today without you.

Epilogue

MID-SEPTEMBER 2015

My eyes opened to the sound of an ambulance. I placed two pillows over my head, trying to block out the sirens. The wails rudely pierced through my pillow fort.

"Fuck you, ambulance!" I said out loud, shoving my pillows back under my head and then, furious, I crawled to the window and gave it the finger.

"I think that will tell it who's boss," my husband quipped. His sleep-filled eyes glared, *you are clinically insane*.

"What time is it anyway? I am so nauseated. I may puke." I lay back down, closing my eyes, trying to ease the rocking seasick feeling that had hit me hard.

"Six fourteen in the morning. Go back to sleep for a bit, my love." He closed his eyes and reached out for me to cuddle.

"Okay," I answered, cuddling him back to sleep.

7:15 A.M.

"Sebastian, I swear these things have gotten so big. I think they are going to burst," I said, sandwiching my boobs in my hands as I rolled over, waking him again. "They're like udders—'milk me, milk me.' Maybe I'll produce Nesquik Chocolate Milk. *Moo-mooooo.*"

"Hmm, let me—. Not a bad thing on the big part," my husband answered, making this an excuse to feel me up.

"Ouch, they hurt!" I screamed and rolled back over, taking the entire blanket with me.

"I was looking for chocolate milk. I had a feeling you were a special cow, that's why I married you. By the way, you are a blanket hog," he said, wrapping his whole body around me.

"I am not a hog, I am a cow. Gosh, do you ever listen to me?" I gave him some "pity blanket" to warm him up.

"Let me see this belly," my husband said, making his way through the blankets and placing his hands on my stomach. "I think I feel something."

"It tickles!" I squealed, jumping out of the bed. "That's my cue to get up."

"I guess I should too." He stretched his right arm into a convenient bicep, the left one following suit.

"Stop flexing," I exclaimed with a laugh, watching him look at his muscle.

He winked. "I'm sorry, it just happens naturally when you are so strong like me."

"Yeah, I hate it when that happens," I mocked, flexing my own non-existent muscles.

Moments later, I heard the shower turn on, and I found myself in the closet picking out something to wear.

I stared at my fifteen-week baby bump in the mirror. It didn't look much different yet—like I had eaten a big meal, a burger or something bloating. I stuck it out to simulate what it would soon be and quickly sucked it back. I see all these pregnant women on the streets sticking their small to big bellies out with pride. And really, why shouldn't they? They look beautiful, and it's an amazing time—a time I once thought wouldn't happen to me. But how come I was still so shy about my growing tummy? Is it the same reason I was still in denial that something wonderful could be happening to me? Is it the fact that I am still recovering from an eating disorder? Maybe.

"Get out of the mirror, Dan!" Sebastian screamed when he spotted me. He had nothing but a towel on and smelled fresh of soap and body lotion. I was in such a trance I didn't realize he was already out of the shower.

"I'm just not sure if I like how this dress looks on me," I said, staring at what reflected back at me. She was unrecognizable. I analyzed her hard. Sebastian's cell phone rang, and he walked into the other room. I watched him leave and then turned back to this person in the mirror.

She had pale skin and huge breasts. Her hair was thick, wild, and long. She was all dressed up and looked professional, maybe even important. But some things were the same as the old her: she had a slight bulge in her midsection and she just wasn't sure if it was going to work. She felt a little insecure, and maybe even...fat.

Boo hoo, you're probably thinking. *You are pregnant, duh— that's why you have a bump.* Quickly, I whacked those *fat* thoughts away because I actually liked this new person staring back at me. She was creating something beautiful—a baby. Her body could do amazing things, like feed that baby and take care of that baby. So she must not be all that bad, either. I walked away with a smile.

FEBRUARY 25, 2016

Lying in the slightly elevated hospital bed with an oxygen mask covering my face, I couldn't help feeling like Darth Vader.

I looked up and saw Sebastian and my dad standing above me. They were trying to act calm, but their forehead wrinkles told another story. I looked down at the wires protruding from the IV coming out of my arm, tracing it carefully with my fingertips and then looked back up at them with a comforting half-smile and flexed my bicep muscle, like Sebastian does, trying to convince them that I was strong and doing fine.

A nurse with straight red hair named Elle hovered to my left side. "Take a deep breath in and bear down," she said in a loud voice. "Take another deep breath and put your chin to chest," she continued, instructing me on how to push effectively. Her hands were gesturing in all directions as she talked. My feet were in the stirrups, ready to start, and Dr. Ng was at the foot of the bed.

As you may have guessed, I was having my baby. Remembering my time with yoga and knack for mixing up lefts and rights, I looked at Elle like a wide-eyed tarsier monkey.

Then I nodded my head up and down even though I didn't know what the heck I was doing. I had asked my doctor if I could practice pushing my baby out so "I would be good at it" (I clearly still had some raging perfectionism to work on). She laughed, because giving birth is something you can't prepare for. Yes, that question actually happened in an attempt to avoid this unknown scary feeling, but with birth I would soon realize that feeling was impossible to steer clear of.

Sweat poured from the top of my forehead. I smelled of vomit from throwing up during the pain of the contractions.

"I think I'm going to throw up again," I whined, feeling so nauseated I could hardly keep my eyes open.

Elle handed me a small puke pan. *Are you kidding?* I thought as I spewed vomit. I had thrown up in my hair, on my hospital gown, and was shaking profusely. That, combined with itchy skin from the epidural, an apparent side effect that had kept me up all night scratching, made my body weary. But it was showtime! And the one thing I knew above all else was that I was strong.

I pushed and pushed and forty-five minutes into it, over twelve hours into labor, I heard my mom announce from the side of the room that she saw a head. Then, with one more push, at precisely 10:21 a.m., I gave birth to a beautiful baby girl. Vivienne was born on February 25th, the fourth day of National Eating Disorders Awareness Week. I consider this more than a coincidence because I owe my life to recovery. She wouldn't be here without me being in recovery. Now, nothing is a better reminder to be strong and to never fall back than my little girl.

EIGHTEEN MONTHS LATER

Baby number two, a girl named Diana after my late grandma, entered the world. She was born a month early, on September 7, 2017—as anxious to get into this world as we were to meet her. She is absolutely beautiful and such a blessing—both my girls are. They have truly changed my world. I am completely enamored with my family of four.

This whole pregnancy was different for me—more challenging in some ways and easier in others. Running after a toddler made this pregnancy go by so quickly, making it easier because I had no time to analyze my changing body and truly self-loathe. Yet it also made it harder because I couldn't rest like I did the first time around. I also didn't exercise as much; maybe ten to fifteen minutes every other day, as my exercise became running after Vivienne. I was exhausted, and my number-one priority was putting my energy into Vivienne and her activities.

The third trimester was rough, with pregnancy side effects that I hadn't experienced the first time around (itchy skin at night, bad headaches/ocular migraines, Braxton Hicks, etc.), and then there was my unrecognizable body on top of that. I came to the realization that I will never love how I look being pregnant, but you know what? That's okay. I would like to make a clear differentiation, too. I struggled with how I looked, but I did practice total self-love in the way I nourished and cared for my body. I was not self-destructing because I was thinking of the beautiful child I was fortunate enough to bear (and the one that was outside my belly, looking at me as a role model). I just think it's important to say that I did struggle with it, so others know it's okay to not feel perfect about your baby bump all the time. It doesn't mean you don't feel lucky and appreciative that you are pregnant or that you are going to relapse. In fact, I am way too happy in my ED-free life to ever look back. Bottom line, I am healthy and how I feel about my third-trimester size is never going to stop me from growing my family—or being the best version of me for them.

I know I will be healthy for my daughters so, in a way, they will always be keeping me honest about my recovery. I never want to hear the words "I am fat" out of their mouths. I never want them to emulate unhealthy eating habits from me. I want them to look at their mommy and see a confident, smart, kind woman. I want them to see that intelligence and a kind heart is what real beauty is. Helping people is what beauty is. Being happy and healthy is what beauty is. The rest is bullshit. I want them to know that bodies come in all shapes and sizes and no one is more perfect than another. I want them to never compare themselves to anyone. I will teach them self-acceptance because no one is perfect. It's the world's greatest farce.

It takes five to seven years for full recovery from anorexia. And *yes*, I do believe in FULL recovery from anorexia, or what I will call *remaining in* FULL for the rest of your life. I am on my way, and I'm determined to be here. I am always on the quick path too—I mean, I am the girl that got engaged after four months! At times, I feel like I am totally recovered already, as I could never imagine, nor would I want to ever go back to that double life. Just to note, it has taken me *time* to get to this place, over six years. I still have a poor body image at times, but maybe, within the next few years, that will disappear as well. Recovery seems to be a waiting game, with *time* being key—for someone with no patience like me, that can be so hard.

My life is so much better without constantly thinking about food. It's not perfect, but that's what I love about it. It's real, raw, and filled with pure happiness and sadness. If you are struggling, you have to know that your happiness is possible, and it comes hand-in-hand with recovery. I never felt joy like I had when I was a child until I was in recovery. I didn't even know that kind of happiness could exist in my adult life. I am not saying that I don't have doubts, but that little voice of anorexia is easily knocked out by my husband's lips against mine, by my making a difference in someone else's life, by my ability to think clearly, by my baby girls.

My advice to anyone struggling to take the leap toward recovery: The longer you live, the more meaning your life acquires. Let yourself live to find it. Now I have so many things to live for. I have a family and a husband. I know no one in this world would love them as much as I do. I want to be around, for them and for me— to experience life with them. To make memories with them. Give yourself a chance to recover, and the meaning will come.

My life has been colorful so far, but I think that color has made me into the strong individual I am today. I wouldn't change a thing. I want to be recovered and happy and help others who are struggling find their FULL as well. I plan to make a life out of it, a FULL life. This is not the end of my story, but just the beginning. To be continued...

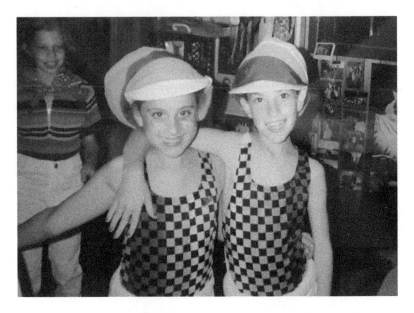

(Above) Camp, with a friend, summer going into sixth grade

(Below) Me at my cousin's wedding, November 2012. I didn't take many pictures during this time.

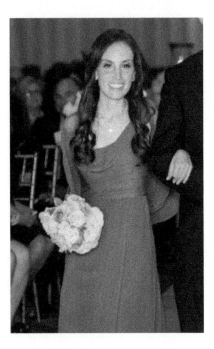

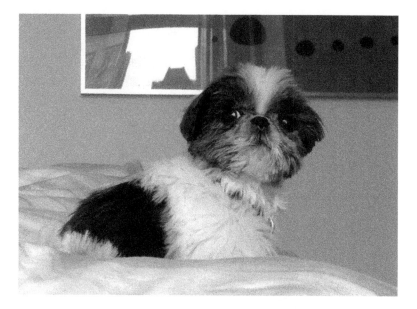

(Above) Teddy

(Below) Me, a year into my recovery, rocking my "Nobody's Perfect" shirt

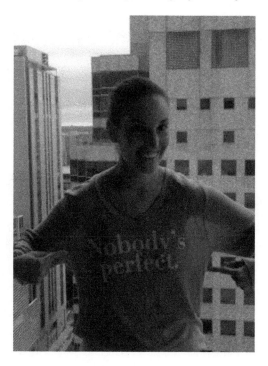

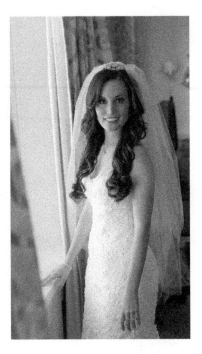

(Above) Wedding ready, October 25, 2014

(Below) NEDA walk with my husband, October 2015

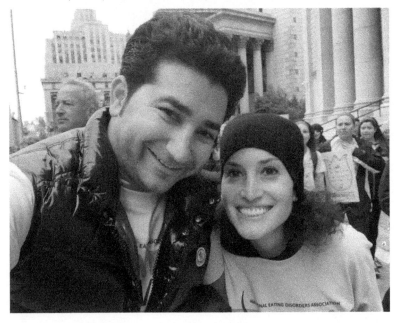

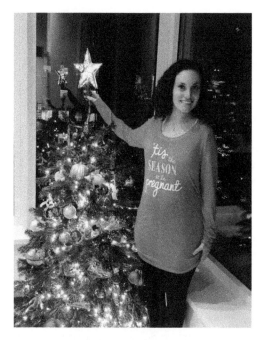

(Above) Thirty weeks pregnant in front of our Christmas tree, December 2015

(Below) My husband, daughter, and me at the NEDA walk 2016

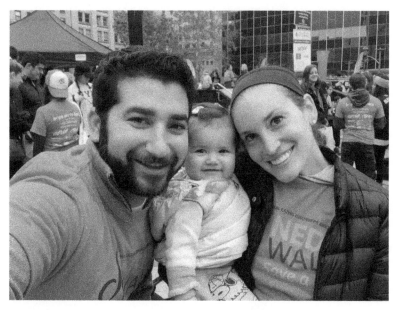

For Potential New Mothers

The moment I found out I was having a baby I was beyond happy—my mind was on a cloud, partying with my friends, the Care Bears. Anybody who longs for a child might feel this, but my joy was infused with such gratitude and relief that it's hard to put into words. I had thought I had completely ruined my body, but once I got my weight back to a healthy BMI and my period became regular, I was able to get pregnant.

I will never forget the day we found out. It was Father's Day, June 21, 2015; we were with my mom and dad for the weekend. I was five days late for my period, but I was spotting, so thought it must be on its way. Sebastian decided to buy a pregnancy test, just because "Wouldn't it be cool if we found out we were pregnant on Father's Day?" *Yes, husband, that would be pretty awesome.*

When we got back to our room, I peed on the stick that would illuminate our fate. Then we sat on the bed waiting for the stupid timer on Sebastian's phone to go off. We had taken these tests before, and when you want to be pregnant *so* badly, that wait is brutal.

Sebastian held my hands in his. "It's still so early. If we don't get pregnant this month, we still have next month and next month. We'll just keep trying." He was the calm and composed to my crazy and anxious. That's why we work.

"I know," I answered, and I did *know* all the sensible jibber-jabber he was telling me, but I was afraid it was going to take a lot of time for me to get pregnant because of all the abuse I'd put my body through. The timer on his phone pinged, and we went into the bathroom, hands clasped together. I could tell by his big grin that the test was positive. I jumped up and down before he could even tell me. I grabbed the test to see it for myself.

"Oh my gosh, we are going to have a baby!" I shrieked. I placed my hands over my mouth in disbelief. *I am having a baby!*

As excited as I was in that moment, once it sank in, there was a part of me that was afraid that the weight gain would jeopardize my recovery. I'd finally found balance in my routines and eating and felt strong in my recuperation, and this was a curve ball. But then there was another part of me, a much greater part, that wanted a baby more than anything and knew, no matter what, I would be okay. I would make sure of it because my baby would need me to be.

Here are some pointers that helped me through my pregnancy that I think could be useful for someone pregnant who is in recovery from eating disorders:

When you are pregnant, you are expected to gain a certain amount of weight. Every time you are at the OB's office, you will be weighed to make sure you are on track. I would advise that you stand backward on the scale and let the professionals track your weight without you knowing what it is. As long as you are on track, that's all that matters. I know people without eating disorders who do this. I know that weighing myself is a trigger, and I took no chances with triggers when it was about the health of my child. That is why standing backward and not knowing my number was a good solution for me.

It is also very important to be up front with your gynecologist/obstetrician about your eating disorder history and past. I was more comfortable emailing my doctor about my history than talking to her in person about it, so that's what I did. It is important to note that I switched gynecologists because Dr. Chang's bedside manner wasn't great for me. When you are having a baby, you are getting intimate with your gynecologist, to put it mildly. You have to feel completely at ease and open with the person who is delivering your baby. I found an obstetrician who fits that bill for me.

The other issue I struggled with sometimes was my actual bump size/physical weight gain, not surprisingly. Sometimes I thought it looked cute, and other times I thought I looked chubby or like a "beluga whale"—more the latter, honestly, which I am not proud of. I was carrying very side to side, so I just started looking pregnant around twenty-eight weeks. I was waiting for "the bump" for so long, and once it came, I was actually not that comfortable with it.

What helped a lot was that I had gotten a great maternity wardrobe that I felt comfortable and confident in. I would suggest everyone get clothes that fit and feel good, especially toward the end of pregnancy! It was helpful to invest in a maternity wardrobe, and it's not a waste of money; I still wear the clothing postpartum. I also plan to have more kids one day, so they can definitely be reused. It's better to avoid all of your old clothes during this time. It can be a sting to your ego when your clothing starts to get tight and can serve as a reminder that you are packing on the pounds.

Let me be real, though: toward the end of pregnancy, every mama-to-be starts feeling huge. From backaches to shortness of breath, it is definitely not a picnic. I remember coming home from a spin class and looking in the mirror and telling Sebastian, "I feel like a sausage," and *I did!* But I think every mother-to-be goes through what I will now call the "sausage" phase of pregnancy—when you feel so big, round, and cylindrical that you think, *Oh shit, I turned into a sausage.* The redeeming moments were when I felt my daughter's kicks, or when she pushed hard on my stomach. Those moments made me realize it would all be worth it, and I was one lucky piece of sausage.

On days when I did feel insecure about my bump, I felt guilty talking about it. If I complained, "I was feeling huge and bad about myself," I would be met with "but you are having a baby." Then I would feel extremely guilty for my feelings, because yes, I was having a baby and I was extremely lucky, but on the other hand, I am allowed to feel not great about myself.

It is ironic that our need to be skinny is dictated by the media and society, but then if we have a fear of getting fat when we are pregnant, it is considered blasphemous and we are thought of as superficial. Addressing any downsides of being pregnant is frowned upon and seen as taboo, but it shouldn't be. I bet you that most mothers-to-be have insecure days and these so-called "irrational fears." We have to start supporting, rather than judging, one another so that we can talk about these normal fears and make one another feel better, instead of holding the feelings in.

Even women who aren't in recovery from an eating disorder worry about their post-baby bodies and getting back to their pre-baby weight, so I knew this was going to be a tricky time for me. Surprisingly, the pull to diet wasn't as prominent as I expected. First of all, I hate unrealistic cultural expectations. I think they are unfair and create so much pressure for women, on top of caring for a newborn! I don't think it's possible that your body will be exactly the same; it has been through so much. Honestly, I like my new body better because it gave me the greatest gift.

With the stress of having a new baby, it is easy to feel, "I am not doing a good enough job" and everything is completely out of control. These times are when the disordered eating thoughts came back into my head, and I had to be vigilant about shutting them down. Wanting a perfect body is hardest to resist when everything around you is so out of control. I had to remember that the size-zero jeans in my closet weren't the key to my happiness; in fact, they made me the most miserable I had ever been. I had to take a step back and realize that I was only obsessing about fat because I felt overwhelmed (balancing working from home and a new baby who needs to eat every two to three hours), and I shut the voices down. In time, when I was getting more sleep, hormones were balancing out, and when I was getting used to being a mother, the pull to diet was far less.

When I wrote about my recovery process earlier, I mentioned that I never saw a nutritionist, and I thank Dr. Attia so much for this. A nutritionist would have put me on a meal plan that would again focus on calories, portion sizes, and all that fun stuff some of us anorexics love to obsessively think about. Dr. Attia told me that no one knows nutrition more than an anorexic, and this is true according to my experience. I could be a nutritionist; I know so much information about how to lose weight, what is healthy, and what is not. Putting me on a plan would be unproductive. I think it may work for some, but for me, it would just put the focus back on calories and not on health. I mean, I would have had a field day talking to the nutritionist, learning more and more to appease my eating-disordered self, but it would keep that little flame of obsession alive.

Out of curiosity, I reached out to Dr. Attia and asked her to clarify her stance on nutritionists in general, because I was wondering why she didn't suggest using one for me, even though she had said it would be useful to some people. I also was curious what she would recommend doing after pregnancy to lose the baby weight. She wrote me an email response:

I think nutritionists are wonderful and can be very useful in the treatment of eating disorders. I initially dissuaded you from consulting a nutritionist because, when underweight, you were preoccupied with many details about eating and I thought you might do better with a single voice working with you on your food choices. Also, at the very start, you were allowing your parents to help supervise your eating and they were well informed (and asked good questions allowing them to remain well informed) about how best to feed you.

I have found that for some underweight folks, nutritional counseling by a dietician may not be necessary. The focus of treatment is on breaking your food rules, allowing you to normalize weight by liberalizing amounts and variety of foods. You knew a great deal about nutritional content; we had to work on helping you to allow yourself to use what you knew!

With this said, some individuals find nutritional counseling to be a very helpful piece of the treatment team, and some clinicians depend on the expertise of a nutritionist or dietician in order to move treatment forward.

As for my other comment about working with a nutritionist during pregnancy or post-pregnancy, I think that a nutritionist has the expertise to keep a close eye on necessary nutrients during these phases. It's not required to consult with a nutritionist, but it could be very useful, especially if you are no longer consulting anyone else about eating or weight issues.

So there you have it.

During pregnancy, I became my own nutritionist in a way, monitoring what was going into my mouth, but in a positive way. I was feeding more than just myself, and that was eye-opening. Pregnancy actually helped me broaden my food freedom within recovery. It made me self-reflect and realize that I still had room to grow. If I was completely honest with myself, there were still some foods I stayed clear of because they were food fears. During pregnancy, I was more willing to let myself try those foods again, like peanut butter, because they were healthy and nutritious for my body and the baby. That rationale really changed my whole outlook. I knew variety and healthy fats were good for my baby, so I pushed myself. Also, when pregnant, you are not allowed to have a lot of foods like deli meat and sushi, so I had to replace these comforts with other foods that I was allowed to have. Everything in moderation, and I was really learning a better balance.

I was also still abusing alcohol and pills to sleep and eat comfortably in certain situations, even in recovery, and being pregnant made me realize that I didn't need these methods as a crutch in my new, recovered life. I went off of Xanax a couple of months before Sebastian and I started trying to get pregnant. I also slowed down the alcohol when we were trying to get pregnant and cut it out completely once I found out I was pregnant. These days, I actually don't drink anymore because, after some reflection, I didn't like what I was using it for. I am still off Xanax and never plan to go on it again. I was replacing one evil with another, and now that I don't have any evils, I feel the best I have ever felt. I like sober life a lot better—I get more done (Exhibit A, this book!). Also, it helps to be fully aware while taking care of little ones. I don't want to miss a moment with my babies. I will never choose to be numb in any way again, so alcohol, pills, bingeing, purging, and starving are all out of my life.

Food & Feelings Journal

The following is a snapshot of the things I found important in recovery. Hopefully it can help you better understand your Maudsley recovery or that of your child or other loved one. I started this journal four days into treatment. The foods I was eating could be used to gain weight, and I gained about seventeen to twenty pounds during this initial period from December to March, but everybody and every body is different. Also, it should be noted, because journals are intended for the writer's therapeutic purposes, rather than literary entertainment, they are necessarily redundant. Therefore, the reader is advised to read or skim only as much as he or she may need for their own benefit.

FRIDAY

Time: 6:15 a.m.
Breakfast: Lydia's Organic Sprouted Cinnamon Cereal and Fiber One mix with milk in a bowl.
How I am feeling: I was not very hungry. I was nervous about my therapy appointment, but I ate the entire bowl. I felt extremely full and exhausted after.

Time: 12:45 p.m.
Lunch: Cream cheese and lox on Mom's special nutritious bread[7] and Dr. Brown's cream soda.
How I am feeling: I shut the door to my and my dad's conjoint office space to block out all the people at work before we ate our lunches together. For some reason, I always feel rushed at work—afraid someone may come in and make a comment about "me actually eating." Yes, believe it or not, people *actually* say that to me now that I am eating—correction, being helped to force-feed myself. I ate it pretty quickly out of fear of those comments. I am finding that just getting the food down as quick as possible is my best method of ingestion these days.

During the meal, my dad called in Marie, our secretary, to retrieve papers on his desk. I was a little annoyed at him and afraid she would make a comment about what I was eating, but she didn't. I felt relieved, but I am still very uncomfortable eating in front of people because honestly, I can't take their comments or the attention it draws to me. It makes me hate myself a little more and makes me feel even more sorry for myself. People think it's okay to continue to jokingly put me down for not being able to do something so natural like eat. My condition is not a choice. I explained this to my dad and he said he understood, the best

---

7   Mom's special nutritious bread, which I dubbed "special" because she was obsessed with using it. It didn't take a team of NASA scientists to figure out. It was fattening but healthy bread, high in calories. Fattening plus high in calories equals Dani Sherman putting on pounds.

someone without an eating disorder can. He probably thinks I am crazy, but I would have to agree with that sentiment. My hands were shaking as I finished my sandwich. Then I went back to work, trying to distract myself from the never-ending dialogue: *You are so fat and worthless, Dani. No one will love you if you gain weight.* It's so hard not to believe it.

Time: 4:09 p.m.
Snack: A whole bag of Nuts 4 Nuts that I got off the street of NY.
How I am feeling: I was still a little anxious because the door was open while I was eating. I feel so much shame when people watch me eat. It's like I failed with each bite, each consecutive chew, and each swallow where I should just *spit it out.* It has become the most humiliating task. I placed the bag of nuts behind my big calculator to conceal them and ate them as I worked. I tried to ignore everything around me, footsteps of people passing, murmurs of voices—but my heart was beating so fast and hard making me cognizant to all of it.

Time: 8:45 p.m.
Dinner: Egg and cheese omelet sandwich on nutritious bread with butter, a cup of hot chocolate with whipped cream, and an oatmeal raisin cookie.
How I am feeling: I felt hungry and tired. I took my medication before dinner to take the edge off. I didn't feel anxious after that, just exhausted. It is easier for me to eat at home than out at a restaurant in front of people. I swear people at other tables look and point at the skeletal girl and judge me—whispering in each other's ears as if it's not obvious because I can't hear them—but, oh yes, I can. I swear my anorexia has given me telepathy. I hear their thoughts like a sixth sense. They pity me as I shake. Maybe it is all in my head, but I see it in people's whispers and stares all the time. After eating, I was a little nauseated. I get queasy almost every night. I think my body is rejecting the food.

Just Some Insight: My medication was 2 mg Xanax and 25 mg Lexapro.
Note: When you have anorexia, and are at low weight, your brain is actually smaller—explaining a tendency for paranoia. If you are an insecure person, you may become more insecure, convinced that everyone is talking about you. I was also "exhausted" because some people get even more tired during recovery than they were before, because their bodies finally have nutrients to repair all the damage caused by starvation and their energy goes toward that.

SATURDAY

Time: 8:30 a.m.
Breakfast: Lydia's Organic Sprouted Cinnamon Cereal and Fiber One mix and vanilla granola mix with milk in a bowl.
How I am feeling: I was tired and feeling not well at all, emotionally, physically—*everything* was bothering me. I ate breakfast and then went upstairs and watched a movie in bed with my mom. It is really weird not doing anything productive without making myself sick—it made me anxious to be honest. At 10:30 a.m., I took an hour nap. I woke up with a puddle of drool on my pillow, but felt a lot better. I took a shower and was

a little bit more awake and ready to start the day. It's hard to be motivated when the day is fully surrounded by food.

Time: 12:45 p.m.
Lunch: Crab cake sandwich on a Kaiser roll and a glass of wine—I ate the whole crab cake sandwich. I also had a glass of Riesling wine.
How I am feeling: I felt very full still from breakfast, but whoever dictates three meals a day fucked me over, because it was time for lunch. We went to a restaurant on the water called the Charter House. I hate going out, especially because of the way I look and the way I shake with each bite. I know it's obvious to an outsider that I have a problem. I have become hyperaware of my hair, bald spot included, and other features I wasn't focused on for the past couple of months prior to getting help. It makes me a little more self-conscious when I am out in public. We took our time eating and had conversations about me as a child. I felt my parents pining for the happy little fluffy-haired girl they once knew. I hope she isn't dead. It ended up being a relaxing lunch—the most relaxed I could possibly be at least with food in front of me. I hadn't had crab cakes since I was little. I wasn't even sure if I liked them when I ordered them, but they were very tasty for fried fatty cakes filled with breadcrumbs and fat. *Did I mention the fat?* I wanted to puke at the thought of what was in my stomach. I would have done anything to take laxatives. I know, I brought up the toilet taboo subject, and the fact that I want to defecate makes me feel even grosser. *You are fat and disgusting.* That sums up how I felt after this meal.

Time: 4:00 p.m.
Snack: Pumpkin muffin and eight ounces of water.
How I am feeling: I wasn't hungry at all, but I knew I should eat it at this time or I would have trouble eating dinner. I knew I had to eat both dinner and this stupid snack too. My mom handed it to me with a look of "don't fuck with me," as I hesitated. I ate it while we were watching a movie, but I had a horrible headache during and after. I think I am allergic to this much food. Scratch that out, I *know* I am allergic to this much food! I even expressed this *concern* to my mom, but she wasn't amused: "Mom, I am allergic to all of this food. It's giving me headaches. Maybe I should see an allergist and get myself tested."
"Shut up, Dan." Gosh where did her sense of humor go?

Time: 9:00 p.m.
Dinner: Egg and cheese sandwich on nutritious bread with butter and eight ounces of water.
How I am feeling: I still had a headache. The only food I thought I could stomach was an omelet sandwich because I was comfortable with it. Why? Because I have eaten it a couple of times before. The more I eat something the less scary it becomes. I took my medication before dinner and didn't feel anxious at all. After eating I was a little nauseated and my stomach hurt.

I went to bed and tossed and turned, waking up in the middle of the night parched. I got up at 3:30 in the morning to get a bottle of water from the kitchen, which was a battle itself because my legs were *so* stiff. I had to sit down at each step to rest them.

By the time I got back upstairs, it was 4:00 a.m. My poor stupid legs were in so much pain. I felt like I had an intense workout from going up and down the stairs one time! *At least you burned calories.* When I got back, I watched TV the rest of the night and massaged my legs. I couldn't help trying to calculate the calories I burned from going up and down the stairs once, and I hated myself for that. Fuck you, voice. I am starting to really doubt if it will ever go away.

SUNDAY

Time: 9:00 a.m.
Breakfast: Lydia's Organic Sprouted Cinnamon Cereal and Fiber One mix and vanilla granola mix with milk in a bowl.
How I am feeling: I was very awake even though I slept badly. I was actually happy it was morning and other people, meaning my parents (my current social life—pathetic), were up. I was ready for breakfast and actually kind of had an appetite. My head was feeling better, which was promising. I ate the entire bowl of cereal.

Time: 2:10 p.m.
Lunch: Spinach and mozzarella pizza—two slices of a small. I also had a glass of pinot grigio wine.
How I am feeling: I felt terrible. We went out with Elizabeth for lunch. My parents thought it would be good for me to see a familiar face. Wrong! I didn't want to see anyone in the state I was in. Especially her. I was upset the entire time. Elizabeth showed up drunk like a beer fish with a shitty attitude and she is roaming free, happy-go-lucky. Life is so unfair. I've done everything that would be considered right and she's done everything so selfishly and wrong. Yet, we both have issues and she gets to live on her own, while I am a twenty-five-year-old failure who lives at home.

I don't think she even knew what was going on with me or cared. She answered my parents' questions, not asking anyone about themselves, which was okay by me since I was in no mood to talk about me either. I was happy to simply remain:
Silent.

Time: 8:15 p.m.
Dinner: Mom's homemade quiche with ham, onion rings, and cheese and eight ounces of water.
How I am feeling: I felt sad and hopeless and questioned if I could recover in general. I had a breakdown before dinner. Seeing Elizabeth made me realize what a failure I was. I didn't want to see her. I didn't want to see *anyone* in the state I was in. Why did my parents make me see her? I keeled down on the floor and started hysterically crying, tears and snot dripping from my nose and red eyes, irritated from rubbing them. I didn't want to eat. I didn't want to feel emotions.

When my parents didn't agree with my protests, I got angry and turned to go upstairs, making it only a couple of steps when my dad swooped me up and carried me back to the kitchen chair, my legs kicking like a toddler's. I fell to the seat next to me, crying until I felt completely weak and defeated. I didn't want to eat; I wasn't hungry. *You are useless. You will never recover. You will just be fat and unhappy.* Why did I have to? My mom rubbed my back.

"If you don't calm down you are going to give yourself a panic attack, Dani." (Four-second thinking pause.) "I am going to have to call Dr. Attia because I don't know what else to do," she said, reaching her own breaking point.

I tried to calm down, but I couldn't.

"Okay, Mom, I am try...trying," I said, breathing hard as tears leaked down my face. I could hardly get the words out. "I am so tired," I said, looking at the slice of quiche in front of me.

"I know you are," my mom answered. Her right hand was on my back as if holding on to me for dear life. I stabbed the quiche with my fork and took a little piece of it into my mouth. Each bite was harder. I wanted to throw it across the room, but I sat there until the plate was completely empty. My hands shook as I finished.

"Happy?" I angrily asked, putting the plate in the dishwasher. My mom didn't look happy. I know she hates seeing me go through this. I then went upstairs to my room and continued crying.

Time: 9:30 p.m.
Snack: One plastic bag of trail mix—attempted to eat: my mom brought it to me. How kind of her? (Obvious Sarcasm Alert!)
How I am feeling: Tired and sad.

MONDAY

Time: 6:30 a.m.
Breakfast: Lydia's Organic Sprouted Cinnamon Cereal and Fiber One mix with milk in a bowl.
How I am feeling: I didn't feel like starting the day. I didn't sleep well from all that transpired the night before. I woke up at 2:30 a.m. to get water downstairs again—legs stiff and pained from the seizure. Going up and down the stairs felt equivalent to running The New York City marathon. And I actually have no desire to ever run that much. Note to self: I really have to start remembering to bring up water the night before because then I won't have to go through this. I got back into bed physically exhausted, but my eyes weren't tired. I tossed most of the night. I had to go to work even though I didn't feel like it. At least it was a distraction from food.

Time: 12:20 p.m.
Lunch: Cream cheese and lox on Mom's special nutritious bread and Dr. Brown's cream soda.
How I am feeling: I wanted to prove to myself that I was going to be okay. I decided not to shut the door to my office today to eat. I wanted to be a normal person without an eating disorder. I didn't want eating to be a secret or a ritualistic thing I was ashamed of anymore. I was ready to take the comments: "You are eating, wow" or "I am happy you're eating." I would say, "Fuck you, I am happy I am eating too." Maybe.

No one came by, and I actually relaxed and had a nice lunch instead of stuffing it down my throat. I still find myself shaking as I put the food into my mouth. My whole body wants to discard it. I sat across from my dad, which was our new routine (at least so far this week). Instead of eating in front of our desks while we did our work, we talked and ate our lunches.

Time: 3:00 p.m.
Snack: Pumpkin muffin and eight ounces of water.
How I am feeling: I felt stuffed from lunch, not hungry. I ate the muffin really quickly because I was nervous who would approach. I felt like I was stuffing the muffin down my throat the way Jughead from Archie comics ate his burgers. All I needed was a big silver crown around my head—oh yeah, and a super amazingly fast metabolism. I should put an ad on Craigslist for one of those.

Well, apparently, I don't have the finesse of Jughead either. This was proven when I started chocking on the muffin, crumbs spewing out of my dry mouth. I chugged a water bottle to try to stop the hacking. I didn't want to draw more attention to myself.

My dad said, "Are you all right?" jumping up from his work chair. *No, you are making me eat so much food*, I wanted to tell him telepathically. Instead I said: "Yes, just needed some water."

He sat back down.

My stomach hurt almost immediately.

Time: 8:00 p.m.
Dinner: Melted American cheese on a cinnamon raisin bagel.
How I am feeling: I felt hungry and tired. I took my medication before dinner to take the edge off. By the time I ate—thank you, 2 mg Xanax—I didn't feel anxious at all and I really enjoyed my meal.

"These are the best bagels, but they are *so* big," I said to my mom, making an observation.

"Yes, they are pretty gigantic," she said, sitting across from me at the kitchen table. She was munching on some boiled chicken with broccoli.

"I feel like we have the deepest conversations at dinners like these," I quipped as I took a bite. I separated the bagel into four pieces. Sectioning the bagel made it easier to conquer. I couldn't help but still have some rituals even while trying to eat during my recovery. I was able to eat it all this way though, and that's what matters right now.

Time: 9:00 p.m.
Snack: Three cups of trail mix (dried fruit, nuts, and M&Ms) and a bottle of water.
How I am feeling: I was really hungry and ate a lot, borderline way too much, of trail mix. I had three whole cups and felt really full after. My stomach bloated out like a beer belly directly after I did the damage. I basically binged, and now I couldn't purge like I used to. I slept terribly. As soon as I lay down, the voices came: *You fat pig, oink oink. You are worthless. Oink oink*. I felt so guilty. I stroked Teddy to try to distract my mind. He was fast asleep, and I could hear his critter-gremlin-like snores

and saw his chest move up and down. At least someone could sleep, I thought, completely frustrated. All I heard was *oink, oink, oink, oink, oink...* all *oink* night *oink* long *oink*.

TUESDAY

Time: 9:00 a.m.
Breakfast: Lydia's Vanilla Crunch Cereal and Fiber One mix with milk in a bowl.
How I am feeling: I didn't feel hungry, but I forced the bowl down or else my mom would get mad at me. I was really thirsty after breakfast and chugged a full bottle of water. I was feeling nauseated this morning probably from last night's binge. Oh, also from the lack of sleep. You became out of control. *You are morphing into a pig and can't stop the transformation. Oink oink, fat ass.* What will happen after I am at my (correction: Dr. Attia's) goal weight? Will I keep on gaining and gaining weight? Will this bingeing still happen? I skipped work today because I felt so bad about myself.

Time: 2:00 p.m.
Lunch: Peanut butter and jelly on Mom's special nutritious bread and Dr. Brown's cream soda.
How I am feeling: My mom wouldn't let me stay in bed. She forced me to get up and go to a movie with her. I ate my sandwich in the movie theater while watching previews. I was still feeling nauseated and like I wanted to close my eyes. I pined for my bed, but now I was stuck at this movie.

Time: 7:00 p.m.
Dinner: Melted American cheese on a cinnamon raisin bagel and twelve ounces of water.
How I am feeling: I had a "feeling bad" day—feeling shitty about yourself all day long and wanting to stay in bed. I took my medication because a "feeling bad" day also consists of drugging yourself to get out of that day as soon as possible. Not to mention, I did have an after-dinner drink or two.

It is common for me to have down days. This is why I started the Lexapro, which takes a combination of weight gain and time to kick in. Dr. Blatter had been trying to get me to take medication for years for my depression, but I was afraid. To be honest, I was afraid I would get fat. But now, why not take it? I was destined to get fat anyway.

My favorite quote on being sad is by comic legend Robin Williams: "I think the saddest people always try their hardest to make people happy because they know what it's like to feel absolutely worthless and they don't want anybody else to feel that way." I would never, ever treat anyone the way I would treat myself.

WEDNESDAY

Time: 6:20 a.m.
Breakfast: Lydia's Vanilla Crunch Cereal and Fiber One mix with milk in a bowl.

How I am feeling: I felt hungrier and a lot better today. That was before I got into a fight with my mom that left me extremely drained. Sometimes I think she believes everything wrong with me is because of her. It's not because of *her* that I am not hungry. It's not because of *her* that I don't have an appetite to eat. It's not because of *her* that I am so "thin." It's because of *me*. It's *my* problem.

I ate my whole bowl in silence. I hate fighting. I usually run away to avoid any sort of confrontation. Cutting, laxatives, or starvation. I like self-destruction—I miss the burn, pain, and hunger. Self-mutilation only involves hurting *my-self* (key word) too. Anything is better than confronting others head-on and telling them how I feel—possibly hurting them. Now, I had to defend myself and piss off someone I love. I feel like this whole ordeal is bad for our relationship, and I wish I didn't have to involve them.

Time: 12:30 p.m.
Lunch: Peanut butter and jelly on Mom's special nutritious bread and Dr. Brown's cream soda.
How I am feeling: Not well. That fight with my mom this morning set me off. I had to shut the door at work to eat lunch. My hands shook terribly. I wanted to cry. I feel like I can't do this—maybe I'll be part of the 20 percent that partially recovers or the 20 percent that never gets better.[8] Maybe I should just check myself in somewhere, save my parents the trouble of my impending failure? But then what if I am part of the latter 20 percent? Would I just live a life full of emergency rooms, eating disorder programs, and mental health clinics? I would rather die than let that happen. I couldn't think about all this shit anymore. All of this self-doubt wasn't helping me eat. Also, peanut butter is a food fear too, and I really should have chosen something else for lunch.

Time: 7:00 p.m.
Dinner: Cheese omelet with butter on Mom's special nutritious bread and twelve ounces of water and some Dr. Brown's soda.
How I am feeling: I was feeling better about everything after talking to my mom about our fight and clearing the air. We both apologized, and like magic, it was as if nothing happened. I ate the whole meal and didn't shake or have trouble eating. Anorexia is definitely a mind game! I talked to my family and didn't really think about the process at all. I just ate slowly and talked, moving steadily through the meal. Bite after bite, that's all it would take. It sounds so easy when I put it like that.

Time: 8:00 p.m.
Snack: Two cups of trail mix (white chocolate chips, cashews, honey-roasted almonds, and mixed fruit).
How I am feeling: I was feeling better about everything, a little more confident that I could do this, and I'd be part of the 60 percent that does recover with treatment, with the help I am getting. I took my meds, ate this in bed, and then watched a movie before I fell asleep. I had a hard time falling asleep again though—damn you, insomnia!

---

8   ANRED. "Statistics: How Many People Have Eating Disorders?" anred.com. Accessed August 22, 2016. https://www.anred.com/stats.html

THURSDAY

Time: 6:10 a.m.
Breakfast: Lydia's Vanilla Crunch Cereal and Fiber One mix with milk in a bowl.
How I am feeling: I actually enjoyed my breakfast. I felt a lot more positive this morning after last night going smoother.

Time: 12:00 p.m.
Lunch: Cream cheese and lox on Mom's special nutritious bread and Dr. Brown's cream soda.
How I am feeling: I ate it with the door shut just because I knew it was probably safer to do that. I was having a good day up to that point, and I didn't want to take a chance that someone would say something that would upset me and ruin it because the last two days were already so rough.

One little comment can send me into a spiral of self-hate. I mean, look what happened yesterday! I hate being so fragile, but I can't help it. I feel like I will grow thicker skin during this recovery process. I will have to and not just because I am going to be putting on weight and that will make me bigger and my skin will probably stretch like Stretch Armstrong—hence, becoming thicker. At least I can have a sense of humor about this whole awful situation!

Anyway, I enjoyed my sandwich in privacy. I am currently feeling a lot better and like everything will work out.

Time: 3:00 p.m.
Snack: A pumpkin muffin.
How I am feeling: I felt very stuffed, like a big round potato, but an ugly kind that Mr. Potato Head would even put on his angry eyes to scowl at. I also felt like I was walking off balance from the pains in my legs from the seizure. I had to pace very slowly and methodically, potato-like, because my legs were so stiff. I felt like my body had a lot of weight, though the scale said otherwise. I was a disgrace to all of potato-kind—an off-kilter-stressed-out-bad-tasting-potato was my current Mr. Potato Head look. I was at risk to be turned into a French fry, a fear food!

I ate the muffin really quickly because I was nervous who would come to the door.

It was tasty, but I felt uncomfortably full. Eating every three hours so heavily is hell on earth for me.

Time: 7:00 p.m.
Dinner: Veggie pizza, a Coke, and eight ounces of water.
How I am feeling: We went out for dinner all the way to Nyack, New York. My dad got his haircut there because he's very loyal to his haircutter, who moved his salon, and my mom asked me(more like kidnaped me) to take the ride with him. We ate pizza at this dive called Turiello's Pizza House & Restaurant, which is known for their delicious slices. I hate to admit, but it was pretty enjoyable in taste even though I couldn't help thinking about all the calories. I almost bit into my fingers from all the shaking! All I could hear was, *all of that fatty grease is going to your already fat ass and jiggly*

thighs! Once I conquered the first bite, it was a lot easier. Or at least I wasn't in as much risk of having fingers as an added pizza topping.

I had a vegetable slice to make myself feel better about eating it, because in my warped mind, vegetables made it healthier. I didn't really touch the Coke, to be honest. I would rather have Diet Coke for many reasons—one being it's zero calories, the other actually being the non-syrupy taste. Overall, it was good to get out of our area.

Time: 8:30 p.m.
Snack: Two cups of trail mix (white chocolate chips, cashews, honey-roasted almonds, and mixed fruit).
How I am feeling: I took my meds, ate this in bed, and then watched some TV before I fell asleep.

I had to start keeping my Food & Feelings Journal in chart form because it was easier for Dr. Attia to track during and after our sessions. She'd be able to look through it during our sessions and get a quick snapshot of my week and then go back after the session to really review what I wrote. Besides the formatting and lack of variation in my diet, she was pleased with my progress.

DAY: Friday		
TIME	**WHAT ATE**	**HOW I FELT**
6:20 a.m.	**Breakfast:** Lydia's Organic Sprouted Cinnamon Cereal and Fiber One mix with a splash of skim milk in a bowl. **Amount:** I ate everything and had half a glass of water.	I wasn't hungry at all. I thought it was from all the trail mix I ate the night before, but I would later find out it was because I was getting my period. When I saw the blood stain in my underwear, I actually smiled. I know, weird reaction, but I was so happy my period came back. It had been gone since April and I want to have babies more than anything one day. If I am going to live, babies would be something to live for, my reason to fight this—right now I don't know if I *really* value myself enough to just fight this for me. I need other motives—future babies are a good one. Also, it means that my body is getting healthier. I don't see my weight gain on the scale, so this is my indication at this point that this is working. That and the fact that Dr. Attia was pleased with me during our first session. But I am feeling the amazing side effects of being a woman with curves: I am tired, crampy, and bloated. *Awesome!*
12:20 p.m.	**Lunch:** Cream cheese and lox on Mom's special nutritious bread and Dr. Brown's cream soda (eight ounces) **Amount:** I ate and drank everything.	I took Midol and was feeling the cramps a little less, but still felt extremely bloated and nauseated. I shut the office door at work because I was feeling insecure about myself as it was. Plus, I was extra sensitive from the raging hormones—making my mood jump around like Mexican jumping beans. *Ay caramba!* I ate the entire sandwich, but I felt very full and gross afterward. *You are so disgusting.* I closed my eyes for a couple of minutes and swayed back and forth trying to ease the nausea after I ate, but it didn't help. I have been getting horribly nauseated after everything I eat. It's like a subconscious physical reaction brought on by my eating disorder voice. But despite the throw-up feeling—gosh I *wished* so hard I could actually hurl instead of just feeling like it—I sucked it up and got back to work.

7:00 p.m.	**Dinner:** Cheese omelet with butter on Mom's special nutritious bread, twelve ounces of water, and some Dr. Browns. **Amount:** I ate and drank everything.	I am not sure if I can participate in treatment anymore. It is just *way* too hard. I know I am very wishy-washy with this, but it's such a struggle. One moment I am feeling good, maybe even *great*, and confident to a degree. The next, I feel like giving up. I had a breakdown before I ate dinner. I was hysterically crying and threw my weak body onto the floor. I felt better after I cried and got the bad feelings out of my system. My mom gave me my medication to calm me down. I felt like sociopath Lisa from *Girl, Interrupted*. I was crazy until calmed down with meds, as a type of restraint. I ate while watching a movie in the kitchen, dazed in thought and dried-up tears. I am not sure if it was hormones or I just doubted myself, but it was enough to make me question everything.
9:00 p.m.	**Snack:** Three cups of trail mix (white chocolate chips, cashews, mixed nuts, and dried fruit). **Amount:** Three half-cup loads in a cup (red plastic cup). I ate it all and went back for refills.	I was in a little bit of a drugged haze, so I started eating handfuls and handfuls of the trail mix. Plus, Xanax sometimes gives me a weird version of the munchies because I become less guarded around food. I was extremely full and uncomfortable after I binged on them. I went to bed feeling so bloated and miserable. *"Did I do that?"* I said doing my best Steve Urkel imitation—imagining myself in multi-colored overalls, glasses and all. I looked down at my empty hands, palms filled with salt. *Dammit* I did.

Note: I had to measure my foods (at least with approximations), with my parents in charge of the measurements, so Dr. Attia would know how much of them I was eating. If I didn't gain weight one week, she could tell me to up the portions of certain foods for the next week.

DAY: Sunday		
TIME	**WHAT I ATE**	**HOW I FELT**
8:30 a.m.	**Breakfast:** Lydia's Organic Sprouted Cinnamon Cereal and Fiber One mix with a splash of skim milk in a bowl. **Amount:** I ate everything and had a full glass of water. The bowl was a standard bowl, and it was filled full with granola and I sprinkled the Fiber One on top.	I felt overtired, sad, and not very hungry. At 4 a.m. I'd gotten out of bed, seeing the light in my parents' room shining bright. I asked what was wrong while scratching, feeding off their nervous energy. *Yes, my skin gets itchy when I am anxious.* "Elizabeth went out and didn't text her mom that she made it home and wasn't answering her cell phone, the doorman phone, or her landline. Her mom and dad are out of town so they pleaded with Dad and me to go to her apartment and check on her. As of this moment, no one has heard from her." My dad went into the city and my mom stayed home with me. *Because they couldn't trust the crazy anorexic to stay at home alone. Maybe she would escape.* After my dad rang the doorbell, Elizabeth appeared discombobulated at the front door. She was okay and alive, but how could she not hear all of those phones? I could picture Elizabeth, brown hair up in a messy bun, eyes dazed and sleep-ridden, irritated that someone came in and woke her up. *I mean, the nerve.* "That girl will never cease to surprise me," I said to my mom as we got the call from my dad that all was fine. "We all have shit," my mom answered as she rolled over, trying to get comfortable in the bed. "True," I said, "like I should talk, right?" I couldn't sleep, and by 8 a.m., we got up and ate breakfast—my poor dad just getting back to sleep in my childhood bed. Afterwards, I went back to my parents' bed and watched TV. I was tired from our chaotic night. I think we all were.

2:30 p.m.	**Lunch:** Slice of whole-wheat pizza with vegetables and two glasses of Riesling. **Amount:** Big slice of pizza pie and two half glasses of wine.	I was hungry but felt fat. I know, what the ED world says: "Fat is not a feeling." Dr. Attia introduced me to this concept. *But how come I feel this way?* How you are physically is not a feeling, but I can't describe how I feel right now any differently. I have gotten to a point where it is hard to separate the eating-disordered voice from my own; they have become one. ED spoke to me every moment, of every hour, of every day. I am working on creating a new voice, but it's not easy to find it. Especially when I can't pinpoint my *real* feelings—angry, upset, irate, mad—gosh, I hate them all! Especially when exploring my feelings creates more pain and more negative thinking. Take today, for instance. My dad commented that my face looked fuller, as in, healthier, and I took it as fat and I wanted to cry. All I heard as I looked at the pizza was: *Don't eat that, your face will get fatter...* After two glasses of wine, I had an appetite and was uninhibited enough to eat the big slice. It was tasty, but I wasn't feeling great about myself, especially because that comment resonated. *I must be getting fat,* is all I can think now. *You see, fat again...*
8:30 p.m.	**Dinner:** Melted American cheese on a cinnamon raisin bagel and a glass of water **Amount:** I had two very large halves of a cinnamon raisin bagel with three slices of American cheese and margarine melted on it, and eight ounces of water.	I felt really worn out. I wanted to eat to get it over with for the night. I took my medications and ate the bagel in pieces. It was delicious, but I felt ready to get into bed as soon as I took my first bite. This process is so tiring and grueling. I think recovery is way harder than being sick, at least emotionally. Both are very tiring ways to live, but when I was anorexic I was able to numb my feelings. Now I feel everything, and it sucks.

9:30 p.m.	**Snack:** One cup of trail mix (Raisinets, cashews, mixed nuts, and dried fruit). **Amount:** One half-cup load in a cup (red plastic cup). I ate the entire cup.	I took it upstairs and ate it while I was watching a TV show to try to distract myself from the fact that I was eating. I fell asleep very soon after finishing. I was exhausted from the day. All I could think about was my face being fuller, and I hated myself for that.

Note: I do not condone all of the drinking I was doing. I was on a lot of medications and that mix is dangerous. I also lied to Dr. Attia about the amount I was drinking. I was sneaking way more at times. Yes, it made it easier for me to eat when I was uninhibited, but sometimes alcohol caused me to be emotional and have meltdowns. It also made it hard for me to adapt to eating without the comfort of drinking, which became like replacing one evil with another. Overall it was counterproductive.

Being in recovery, for a while now, I have engaged in more healthy habits like spinning and writing as coping mechanisms. I don't miss drinking at all, and know that I can eat in every situation without it. If I am feeling uncomfortable, more booze or popping a Xanax is not the answer; talking it out with my support system or writing about it until I feel better is.

DAY: Monday		
TIME	**WHAT I ATE**	**HOW I FELT**

6:30 a.m.	**Breakfast:** Lydia's Berry Good Sprouted Cereal and Fiber One mix with a splash of skim milk in a bowl.
	
	Amount: I ate everything and a glass of water. The bowl was a standard bowl and it was filled with granola and I sprinkled the Fiber One on top.
		I felt rested and ready to start the day. I got a good night's sleep last night. I wasn't awoken by any unexpected surprises. I talked to my mom while eating and waited for my dad to get ready for work per usual. He has his morning routines: checks his emails, showers, shaves, and suits up like Barney Stinson on *How I Met Your Mother*.
		
		  I am really fast in the morning—like the furry hippity-hoppity hare. I am ready for work with so much time to spare (rhyming not intentional). I am not approved to do anything physical right now, which is actually okay with me because my body still hurts so much from the seizure. My body moved in ways I never thought possible. It was like I stuck my finger in an electric socket! *Zap!* Then it shorted out and every limb went in different directions. The aftermath doesn't feel too good as anyone could imagine.
		
		  Anyway, I usually use the extra time to watch TV, write in this journal, or sleep after eating. I never spend time on my hair or makeup. My mom encourages me to put lipstick on, but besides that, I don't see the point in getting so done up. I blend in better without makeup. I don't want to draw attention to my "full face." I also wear a baggy uniform every day. With my body changing, I need to conceal the growing fat around my frame. I wear tights with a long red sweater or a long black sweater.
		
		  I petted Teddy as I waited today. He was lying on my long black sweater, almost blending in.

11:55 a.m.	**Lunch:** Cream cheese and lox on Mom's special nutritious bread (whole grain) and Dr. Brown's cream soda (eight ounces). **Amount:** I ate and drank everything.	I felt anxious and a little angry. Those are actual feelings! My dad was pressuring me to eat early so I would have more of an appetite when we went out for dinner later. I was trying to figure out where we were going, and he got frustrated and yelled at me. He had other things that he needed to worry about, "much more important things" and I was bringing up "bullshit" details in my recovery plan. *When was I going to be able to choose my own foods? When could I stay in the house alone? What did he think?* I hate that I care about this crap, but I need to plan ahead. I don't blame him for getting frustrated. After all, obsessing about these things doesn't make sense to a non-eating-disordered individual. After he yelled at me, I felt bad about myself and still do. I don't want to live with my parents anymore. *He thinks you are worthless and so annoying.* I want to go back to my apartment, to independence, to anorexia even. We never really fought, anorexia and I. I feel like anorexia was a big part of my identity. I don't know who I am without it. It's been too long. I feel so out of control in every aspect of my life.
3:00 p.m.	**Snack:** Oatmeal raisin cookie and eight ounces of water. **Amount:** Cookie was the size of my palm.	I was very full, and my stomach hurt, but I ate it anyway so my dad wouldn't get more upset. I was already stressed enough; I didn't need him disciplining me anymore. *He hates you.* I think the voices will always be there.
7:30 p.m.	**Dinner:** Two slices of pizza. **Amount:** Two full slices of pizza.	I had a breakdown after dinner. I binged straight from dinner to the snack after dinner. See below.

7:45 p.m.	**Snack:** Three cups of trail mix (Raisinets, cashews, mixed nuts, and dried fruit). **Amount:** Three half-cup loads in a cup (red plastic cup). I ate the entire cup each time.	I was extremely full and broke down from the stress of the day and all that I ate in a short period of time. I had such bad remorse. I wished I didn't eat it all, but I binged and couldn't stop. My mom tried to comfort me, but I just wanted the day to be over. I wanted everything to go away, including me. I turned bright red and was wheezing, I was crying so hard. I flung myself to the floor in a fit of rage. My mom came down to the floor after me, trying to calm me, and embraced me. She didn't know what to do. "I am going to have to call Dr. Attia, you are going to have a panic attack," she threatened. *Again with that?* I thought.
		I insisted that I would be okay and calmed myself down. I wanted all that I ate to come out *so* badly. *Get laxatives, you fat ass!* I wanted to be empty. I know that laxatives don't control weight loss and by the time they act on the large intestine, most foods and calories are already absorbed by the small intestine. Meaning it is really not that effective. However, it makes me feel thin. Even if it is water loss and wastes from the colon, it is something! It makes me feel a little better, especially after a binge like this. I hated that I couldn't help thinking about them.

Note: Eating is going against everything you stand for when you have an eating disorder. Out-of-control eating without compensation would make me so flustered that I would break down. It was like a demon would take over my body; I couldn't handle it.

DAY: Tuesday		
TIME	**WHAT I ATE**	**HOW I FELT**
9:00 a.m.	**Breakfast:** Lydia's Vanilla Crunch Sprouted Cereal and Fiber One mix with a splash of skim milk in a bowl. **Amount:** I ate everything and a glass of water. The bowl was a standard bowl and it was filled with granola and I sprinkled the Fiber One on top.	I woke up feeling a lot better. I took a shower, washing away my bad feelings from the binge, and ate breakfast. I was hungry and let my mom pour the cereal into the bowl without saying anything about the amount she poured like I usually did. *And* boy I had to hold my tongue, because it was hard for me to remain tight-lipped. Unfortunately, my mom is still in charge of making every meal for me because "I can't be trusted with portion sizes yet," according to Mom and Dad, Dr. Attia, Dr. Blatter—basically the whole team. Hoping that will change really soon. We had a nice light conversation at breakfast. "What are we doing today?" I asked her, as I put a spoonful of cereal into my mouth. "Probably go out for lunch somewhere," she said, sipping her morning coffee out of a blue Disney mug. I couldn't believe she was thinking about lunch already. It made me want to hurl. "Smells good, wish I liked the taste of coffee," I said watching her sip. "Don't worry, you don't need another bad habit, Dan." "Touché, Mom, touché."

1:45 p.m.	**Lunch:** Grilled cheese sandwich with tomato on onion bread and a glass of water. **Amount:** I ate and drank everything. It was the size of a burger, but was grilled cheese and tomato.	We went to the Cupping Room in Soho. I was in a good mood; as good as you can be while trying to overcome an illness. The crowd was young, the friends-and-couples-who-brunch crowd, and immediately I felt uncomfortable and wanted to cover my face, hide in a corner, or crawl into the nearest hole like a mouse. I didn't want to run into anyone I knew in the condition I was in. I scanned the room, completely paranoid. *You are a failure and everyone should judge you. They have relationships, spouses, and live on their own, while you have nothing!* I twiddled my fingers while we waited for a table. I no longer knew how to eat in public. I usually played with the food on my plate while taking sips of a drink. I rarely knew if I was eating politely. The manners I'd learned when I was young were a faint memory. Which fork was for appetizers and which was for the main course? So many rules. Countess Luann of *Real Housewives of New York City* etiquette fame would have a field day with me. I could picture her seated across the table, plugging her book, of course: "Pick up *Class with the Countess*, dahling, it will teach you everything you need to know." "Sure thing, dahling," I'd respond. To my relief, we ended up in a back corner. We had a nice lunch because I had my own private sanctuary to hide in and eat the way I felt comfortable, hoping that the voices would finally leave me alone. They didn't.
5:00 p.m.	**Snack:** Oatmeal raisin cookie and eight ounces of water. **Amount:** Cookie was the size of my palm.	I ate a cookie while we were watching *Homeland*. The cookie was soft and flavorful, and *Homeland* is an amazing show. We, my dad and I, are borderline obsessed right now. It is a nice distraction from what is going on in my life. At least I am not falling in love with a terrorist. Thank you, Carrie Mathison, for making me feel a little better about my own life and putting things into perspective!
8:00 p.m.	**Dinner:** Cheese omelet with butter on Mom's special nutritious bread (whole grain), eight ounces of water, and some Dr. Browns. **Amount:** I ate the whole sandwich.	I wasn't very hungry and opted for something that would be easy to get down. It was good, and afterwards I was exhausted. I have formed food patterns even in this weight-gaining process. I can't eat just anything, and it worries me. I crave the sameness. *Monotony, oh how do I love thee? Let me count the ways like Elizabeth Barrett Browning. Will I ever not love thee... even after death?* (Sonnet ED voice) Please say no!

Note: I used to stand over my mom and judge the amount of milk she poured into my cereal. If she poured too much milk, I wouldn't want to eat it because that meant more excess calories. It made me feel better watching the cereal to know what she put into it.

Eating out at places where I could potentially run into someone I knew freaked me out. I was not proud of where I was in my life. I wasn't proud of how I looked. I didn't want to see anyone. Also, as an anorexic, you develop strange ways of eating. I had suffered on and off with anorexia and bulimia since I was young, so I never developed proper ways to eat certain foods simply because I never had them before or ate them mostly in private with rituals—not manners dictating how I ate. I became insecure that I wasn't eating politely, but my mom would just tell me, "I don't care how you are eating it; I am just happy you are eating."

DAY: Wednesday		
TIME	WHAT I ATE	HOW I FELT
6:30 p.m.	**Breakfast:** Lydia's Vanilla Crunch Sprouted Cereal and Fiber One mix with a splash of skim milk in a bowl. **Amount:** I ate everything and a glass of water. The bowl was a standard bowl, and it was filled with granola and I sprinkled the Fiber One on top.	I woke up this morning at 5:40 a.m. I was dripping sweat—I soaked all the way through my sheets and blanket, a puddle forming the outline of the shape of my body. My hormones have been outrageous. I think that they are trying to regulate. When my mom was blow-drying my hair, hot heat blowing on my scalp and into my face, I almost passed out and had to lay down, body pressed on the cold marble tile in my parents' bathroom, ready to sing the dingle dangle dingle song. I ate the entire bowl of granola. I was feeling a little nauseated and dizzy, so I forced it down, wanting to avoid any possibility of fainting. How could I be almost fainting when I am eating more than I have in my entire twenty-six years of life?
12:30 p.m.	**Lunch:** Peanut butter and jelly on Mom's special nutritious bread (whole grain) & Dr. Brown's cream soda (eight ounces). **Amount:** I ate and drank everything.	I shut the door and had a relaxing ten-minute break. I took a bite of my sandwich while checking my email. I savored each bite like when I was in third grade at sleepaway camp. I love the taste of peanut butter, the gooey, salty, peanut taste. I chewed up the sandwich in small bites and swooshed it in my mouth from side to side. I'd closed the door because I didn't want anyone to see my weird eating habits. *You will never get rid of your rituals. You will just be fat and fucked up instead of skinny and fucked up.* I then felt an overwhelming sadness. What if the vicious voice of ED is right? Today is clearly Wondering Wednesday—*so many questions!*

3:00 p.m.	**Snack:** A bag of NY Nuts 4 Nuts and eight ounces of water. **Amount:** A packet of them. I ate them all and sipped on the water.	I snacked on them while working from 3 to 4 p.m. I was hiding them behind my big calculator so no one would say anything. My parents got them for me because I used to love them when I was little. I smelled their strong aroma with nostalgia—memories of walking the streets of Manhattan. These nuts and FAO Schwarz defined New York for me as a small child—as well as my dad's yellow taxicabs of course. I would beg my parents to get me a package of them. Now, they would beg me to eat them. Boy, things have changed.
7:30 p.m.	**Dinner:** A piece of Mom's homemade quiche. **Amount:** I had a big piece; it is made with ham, cheese, onion rings, and Pillsbury dough.	I had a piece of quiche before my parents went out for dinner with their friends. My mom used to make it for my dad and me during the holidays. It was one of my favorite things, a homemade guilty pleasure. I knew this was a "bang for your buck" item too, so I wouldn't have to eat a lot of it. I remember when I used to binge on this quiche during my junior and senior years of high school. Half the pie would go missing, and no one would say anything. Where did they think it went?
8:15 p.m.	**Snack:** Two cups of trail mix (Raisinets, cashews, mixed nuts, and dried fruit.) I also had a Nutter Butter cookie. **Amount:** Two half-cup loads in a small glass. I ate the entire cup each time. I also had a Nutter Butter cookie.	I snacked on them because I felt hungry, not because I was supposed to *(go me!)*, while watching TV in my room with Teddy. I fell asleep a little after my parents got home, like I'd been a little girl again waiting up for them because I was afraid something awful would happen to them. I would stay up talking to our babysitter, talking her poor ear off, until I would hear the alarm beep, my signal that they were home and safe. I always had this feeling of impending doom, even as a little girl. I could never enjoy anything, and I almost felt guilty when I did.

Note: A "bang for your buck" food item is something small and caloric that will be as much as eating something that is big and not as high in calories. If I were not hungry, this would be a great meal option.

DAY: Thursday		
TIME	**WHAT I ATE**	**HOW I FELT**
6:20 a.m.	Breakfast: New granola called muesli and Fiber One mix with a splash of skim milk in a bowl. **Amount:** I ate everything.	I am never really hungry for breakfast, but it was good. I felt tired though. This process drains me like open apps drain my iPhone battery.
12:30 p.m.	**Lunch:** Cream cheese and lox on Mom's special nutritious bread (whole grain) and Dr. Brown's cream soda (eight ounces). **Amount:** I ate and drank everything.	I love cream cheese and lox. It's Jewish soul food. I ate it in front of my computer. It was a busy day. I don't shake anymore. My dad pointed it out to me, and I looked down at my hands to see that it was true. It made me feel good, like I was at least getting more comfortable around food. Maybe I don't feel myself getting better at times, but my body does.
7:00 p.m.	**Dinner:** Chicken and pine nuts and chicken fried rice with duck sauce on it and a Dr. Brown's cream soda (eight ounces). **Amount:** I ate and drank everything. **Snack:** I also had two cups of mixed nuts in bed.	I was starving. I hate that I am getting hunger cues back. The doctors say I can't trust them yet though. When a body is malnourished, it wants to conserve as much energy as possible and, unfortunately, that includes not sending hunger cues. At the same time, a starving person's fullness cues can also be out of whack. While it takes someone who eats meals consistently about twenty to thirty minutes to feel full, a person who is malnourished or restricting their food intake can feel full after only a few bites because their stomach anticipates that they aren't going to be fed or are going to be fed only a small amount.[9] This is why I am not trusted yet, and I still have to eat on a schedule like this. Also, I am nowhere near my goal weight, whatever that is. I had a lot of computer work today, and my eyes were burning and raw, making them feel heavy. I went straight to bed after I ate even though it was pretty early and fell right to sleep.

I jotted down some questions for my next session with Dr. Attia because I was getting frustrated with not knowing anything. I felt like I was in the dark a lot during this process, and my personality type is *need-to-know*. These are the questions I wrote down, with a summary of the responses:

Question: At what target weight can I start living on my own? And at that weight, will the medicine work? Why *that* number?

9   Cielo House. "Understanding Hunger and Fullness," Cielohouse.com, Jul 29, 2014. Accessed August 25, 2016. https://www.cielohouse.com/understanding-hunger-and-fullness/

Answer: It seemed like around one hundred pounds was my personal target number to start living at home, but it wasn't just about a number. Antidepressants only start working when weight is restored and eating becomes more under control. To start getting some independence back, I would have to be laxative-free and show signs of really recovering. It was way too early in my recovery when I asked this question for the first time. I still had a long road ahead. If I continued improvement in my behaviors, weight, etc., I would be rewarded with time on my own at my apartment, have permission to exercise, and so on.

Question: Are night sweats normal? My period stopped the day before, so I don't think it was that—I woke up completely drenched. I felt like I was going to pass out when my mom was blow-drying my hair the morning after the night sweat.

Answer: It was my hormones regulating. They were trying to balance out after being shut off for so long. This was completely normal. Unhealthy eating styles can lead to changes in reproductive hormones, which are responsible for maintaining regular periods. As a result, some women will have irregular periods, some will stop having them altogether, and some may suffer infertility. This is the body's response to try to save energy and prevent reproduction in somebody who is starving. Hormones will return to normal levels once eating is back to normal. My hormones were trying to regulate back to normal, and the surge in hormones is what caused me to almost faint.[10]

Question: Is there some kind of support group or outpatient weekend program I should or could join? (I didn't ask this question after all, because I was still too afraid. I think this is so smart for others going through recovery because I felt so alone in my recovery when I could have had people around me going through the same thing.)

---

10 You and Your Hormones. "Eating disorders and hormones," yourhormones.info, updated October 24, 2013. Accessed August 25, 2016. http://www.yourhormones.info/topical-issues/eating-disorders-and-hormones/

DAY: Friday		
TIME	**WHAT I ATE**	**HOW I FELT**
6:30 a.m.	**Breakfast:** Muesli and Fiber One mix with a splash of skim milk in a bowl. **Amount:** I ate everything.	Not hungry. I had a stomachache as well. I didn't sleep from 1:30 to 3:45 a.m. and was up watching television. I had to get up at 5:40 a.m. to get ready for the day. I was pretty tired, but my nerves kept me up. I was nervous for my appointment with Dr. Attia. I am always nervous that I won't do good enough with my weight gain or food choices one week and everyone will give up on me and send me away to a residential treatment center. *You are a burden. You deserve to be sent away.* That's all I hear. Constantly. On a side note, my legs are finally getting better from the seizure. For a while I was afraid that they were going to be lead bars forever, but that doesn't seem to be the case. I am going up and down the stairs with much more ease now. To think I am going to ask about working out at this upcoming session while I just started being able to go up and down the stairs without pain. I won't mention that part.
12:00 p.m.	**Lunch:** Cream cheese and lox on Mom's special nutritious bread (whole grain) and Dr. Brown's cream soda (eight ounces). **Amount:** I ate and drank everything.	I felt a little pressured to eat at noon by my dad because we were going out for dinner on the earlier side. I was hyped up with anxiety since I had a lot of work to catch up on and things to accomplish and then ON TOP OF THAT my dad was like "*Eat eat eat*" or at least that's what I heard; and all I wanted to do was scream *Ahh ahh ahhhhh.* I closed the door, trying to calm myself, and my dad and I had a quick lunch with NY1 on TV in the background, which was a nice distraction. I asked my mom to make this meal for me. I usually ask her to make my lunch and put it in a brown bag like when I was in elementary or middle school. Something is comforting for me about a brown-bagged lunch—maybe it is the nostalgia of it. I am not ready to order in on my own yet. There are too many choices. I find it overwhelming. Plus, this way I know the size of what I am getting, what exactly it is, and can mentally prepare to eat it. Oh, and by "on my own," I mean my dad is monitoring me even though he doesn't have a clue about what constitutes a low- or high-calorie meal. This is a man who thinks strawberry shortcake is healthy because it has strawberries in it! He does report back to my mom though, so I can't easily trick him.

| 7:15 p.m. | **Dinner:** Three slices of an individual vegetable pizza pie.

Amount: I ate half of a big individual thin-sliced pizza. It had broccoli, carrots, mozzarella cheese, and tomato. | We went out for an early dinner at this quaint red-brick "Three Little Pigs"-type building that doubles as a restaurant, serving Italian food. I wanted to see if I could find the third and smartest pig. Nope. The big bad wolf must have gotten to him "by the hair of his chinny chin chin." If there was Italian pork on the menu, I knew why. *Oh well.* Anyway, it had a nice fireplace in the corner, giving us our own tiny shining sun. I could hear it crackling as it burned almost at the same beat as my hungry, grumbling stomach.

My mom suddenly had a terrible bellyache and ran to the bathroom. My dad received important news from work and was distracted and on the phone texting. He wouldn't tell me what it was about. I felt like I was out for dinner alone, which is daunting for a recovering anorexic, but then my dad wanted me to edit an email, so I finally found out what it was all about. Still, this dinner was ridiculous. It fell apart.

I suggested we leave to make my mom more comfortable because she kept going back to the ladies' room. My mom insisted she was fine, but eventually agreed she would rather be in her own bathroom. Duh, doesn't anyone who has a bad stomach feel that way! And, trust me, I would know more than anyone. After my dad finished his chicken noodle soup appetizer, we took our main courses home. I didn't mind at all.

When we got home, I ate with my dad in the kitchen, while my mom was sick upstairs. I was jealous that my mom got to skip the meal *and* was getting sick to her stomach at the same time. I hate to admit that. *I miss feeling empty.*

Then while we were eating the rest of our dinner in the kitchen, my dad kept repeating how thin the slices of pizza were, making me feel a lot of pressure to eat more than I was hungry for—like I wasn't doing good enough to appease him. I think he was trying to encourage me to eat more, but his way was making me feel bad. *You are a failure.*

I felt really full and tired by the time I was done eating. We went upstairs to check on my mom and she was okay. She was lying in bed, exhausted—the usual aftermath of a bad stomach. *Don't you wish you were your mom right now?* I heard in my head. Oh, I did. More than anything. |

DAY: Saturday		
TIME	**WHAT I ATE**	**HOW I FELT**
7:45 a.m.	Breakfast: Muesli and Fiber One mix with a splash of skim milk in a bowl. **Amount:** I ate everything.	I really like this mix, but it's breakfast and, *surprise,* I am not hungry. I ate with both my mom and dad—meals have become so "family dinner" formal with everyone sitting at the table together. It wasn't *anything* like it was growing up. Maybe this was making up for that. I was feeling very bloated and extra uncomfortable in my skin. I wanted to rip it off and hide under it. I wished I were a turtle that could retract into my shell. All I wanted to do was stay in the house in my pajamas and rest with Teddy. I didn't want to go out and do anything, but my parents forced me. I don't get why I can't have a day to myself—a day off from everything! *That's because they don't trust you and probably never will,* I thought, and became increasingly angry. *What's the point of trying if no one will ever trust you anyway? All you need are some laxatives and you won't feel bloated anymore.* Damn you, voice! Damn. Everyone. And. Everything.
2:00 p.m.	**Lunch:** Grilled cheese on challah bread and eight ounces of water. **Amount:** I ate and drank everything.	We went to a fancy diner in the city that I never had been to. Let's be real, my time in the city was never spent checking out different trendy restaurants—I had only been to a handful of restaurants even though I had been living in New York, a foodie's mecca, for seven years. I resented my parents for making me leave the house. I was in a bad mood, not really talking to anyone, and I sure as hell did not want to eat. I wanted to be at home, in bed, wrapped tightly under the covers, Ted at my side. I ate the sandwich and felt extremely anxious afterwards. I felt the food creep into my pores, increasing my stomach fat content. *You are so fat.* I felt the fat increase in my cheeks, thighs, kneecaps— yes, you *can* have kneecap fat! It attacked me at all angles. It was a terrorist, and I was its target. I wanted to scream and instead was acting disconnected, and to be frank, a little bitchy. "Dani, what do you want for lunch?" Dad asked, trying to be considerate, knowing I would rather be *anywhere* but under their watchful eyes. I shrugged, pouting and sulking. This was me all day. I was a *real* pleasure to be around.

| 10:00 p.m. | **Dinner:** Cheese omelet with butter on Mom's special nutritious bread (whole grain), eight ounces of water, and some Dr. Brown's cream soda.

Amount: I ate the whole sandwich.

Snack: Sixteen animal cookies. | I was absolutely exhausted. My parents still don't trust me to make and eat my own dinner, so I waited until they got home to eat. Trust seems to be the buzzword of the day. I think if I were playing a drinking game with that word, I'd be completely plastered right now. I find it ridiculous that they don't trust me. I hadn't done anything wrong for them *not* to trust me. Two more shots in the last two sentences. This may get fun for me!

   On the other hand, it was difficult for them too, so I just did what they wanted me to do and ate when they got home. I didn't say anything about the time because I didn't want to fight and a part of me was happy that they went out and had fun. *You take away all of their fun. You are a succubus of fun.*

  I was exhausted because I took my medication at 9 p.m. not knowing they were going to be home so late. I went to sleep right after I ate. The food probably was going to sit in my stomach all night. You are going to gain weight faster—oink, oink, oink. AHHHHH stop it. Shut up! Please. |

DAY: Sunday		
TIME	**WHAT I ATE**	**HOW I FELT**
8:00 a.m.	**Breakfast:** Lydia's Vanilla Crunch Sprouted Cereal and Fiber One mix with a splash of skim milk in a bowl. **Amount:** I ate everything and had half glass of water. The bowl was a standard bowl, and it was half full of granola and I sprinkled the Fiber One on top.	I felt bad for how I acted yesterday. I showered and took Teddy outside into the cold for a walk. The fresh air felt good, clearing my lungs from the dirty anorexia toxins. *Maybe I could freeze this disease out*, I thought, opening my mouth a little wider, inhaling the cold air. I made my dad and myself breakfast, and we ate together at the kitchen table. This was the first time I made myself breakfast, which felt good. I felt like I had some control back. I got to choose how much milk and granola. I didn't put less than what my mom puts in it either, scout's honor. I wasn't going to mess with my own recovery after yesterday being so rough. Today had to be different. I had to be strong. My mom got mad when she woke up and found out that I made breakfast without her. She was sleeping though! My dad vouched that I poured a good amount of cereal and milk. She then changed her attitude and was okay with it. I was bothered that she didn't believe me and needed a verbal confirmation from my dad, but I let it go. I wasn't in the mood to play the *trust* drinking game again today.

| 2:00 p.m. | **Lunch:** Cheese and tomato omelet on bread with two glasses of Riesling wine.

Amount: I had two big pieces of toast with the cheese/tomato omelet between the slices. | We had my parents' friends from North Carolina over. They were going to stay with us for a couple of days. *They will figure you out. They will know how fucked-up you are by the end of their visit.*

We went out for lunch at the Charter House because my parents' friends like boats, so they thought it would be nice to eat by the Hudson River. Plus, it has a beautiful view of New York City. I was nervous because: (a) It was a buffet-style lunch, and (b) I usually got the crab cake sandwich when we went here for lunch in the past, but now, in recovery, that wasn't an option for Sunday brunch. Just this ginormous buffet.

We scanned the buffet before we sat down, and it seemed okay: an omelet maker, French toast, pizza, then some turkey, pasta. *So* much food—and every cuisine! I generally feel uncomfortable around buffets, but I didn't want to make it into a big deal or draw attention to myself. I chose a cheese omelet sandwich for lunch because my mom makes it for me a lot, and I know I can handle eating it in front of people. I then accompanied it with two glasses of wine and felt *much* better. Since everyone else in the buffet piled their plate with food, it made me feel out of place that I only had the omelet sandwich. I mean my dad had breakfast, lunch, and dinner all in one meal! And his stupid joke as he patted his stomach, "It all goes to one place anyway." I fake laughed and chugged the rest of my wine. I don't think I could *ever* do that.

I also can't mix different foods. I can't have a breakfast food with a lunch food; it just doesn't make sense to me. I like to have one solid cuisine type. It makes me feel better and any other way is the equivalent of nails on a chalkboard. I shake, cringe, and just want to scream *ah, ah, ah.*

My mom later told me she saw me shaking a little before I ate, but it wasn't noticeable unless you knew *my problem* and were looking for it. I was a little taken aback because I thought I came across confident and normal. In terms of feelings after the meal, I felt fine. *Ha, don't lie; you felt terrible. You are so weird. You will never fit in anywhere.* |

| 8:00 p.m. | **Dinner:** Melted American cheese on a cinnamon raisin bagel and eight ounces of water.

Amount: I had two very large halves of a cinnamon raisin bagel with three slices of American cheese and margarine melted on it.

Snack: One cup of trail mix. | I felt tired and wasn't really hungry, but I ate the super-sized bagel anyway—like I had a choice! I felt even more bloated afterward. I talked to my parents' friends about their grandkids, etc. They soon after FaceTimed in and the kids were absolutely adorable. One, Sara, was a little girl with beautiful blonde hair and freckles peppering her little nose and around her blue eyes. They called saying goodnight to their grandparents before they went to bed. *How cute? You will never have that. You are too fucked-up.* She made me smile, like a real authentically happy smile, for the first time in a while. The kind of smile only the sweetness of a child could produce. The kind of smile I forget exists way too often. |

DAY: Tuesday		
TIME	WHAT I ATE	HOW I FELT
6:30 a.m.	**Breakfast:** Muesli and Fiber One mix with a splash of skim milk in a bowl. **Amount:** I could not eat anything.	I couldn't eat anything. I got sick to my stomach in the early morning around 2 a.m. The last time I got sick was 5:30 a.m. I had a horrible pain in my stomach, followed by some gurgles and an explosion, volcanic like. I felt nauseated at breakfast and couldn't eat. "I can't eat," I said in protest, pushing the bowl of cereal away. "I really don't feel well," I added as I lay down on the kitchen chairs. "Then you shouldn't go to work," my mom retorted, voice quivering slightly. "No, I'll be fine," I answered, closing my eyes. "I am not happy," were the last words I heard in mumbles under my mom's breath as she angrily walked off. She wasn't happy I refused to eat. She wasn't happy about a lot of things. She thought that if I could go to work, I should be able to force it down. She thought I was using my stomachache as an excuse. *She wasn't entirely wrong, but who wants to eat when they are getting sick to their stomach?* Probably no one. Definitely not a recovering anorexic. Lucky for me, I was too nauseated to care about how she felt.

| 1:00 p.m. | **Lunch:** Peanut butter and jelly on Mom's special nutritious bread (whole grain) and eight ounces of water

Amount: I ate the whole sandwich. | I was still not feeling well. I felt a lot better, but it was hard to eat. I forced it down. I ate with the door closed while chugging water. I was thirsty and dehydrated from my sensitive stomach. I was annoyed because my mom called my dad to check if I was able to eat lunch.

"Did she eat, Mark?" I heard, blaring on my dad's speakerphone. Clever move, Dad.

He responded, "No," even though I told him I was going to eat in a little because I wasn't hungry when he was having his lunch.

"I hear you! Your husband put you on speakerphone. And Dad, I told you I was going to eat in a little!" I screamed, face getting red from anger mixed with frustration.

I was frustrated at my mom for feeling the need to ask my dad and not me about my eating. I called her and told her that if she had a question, she *should* ask me directly and added that it's not a normal question to ask if someone ate lunch—I reversed it to her. She agreed. To her credit, though, this is not a normal situation.

My dad also doesn't listen to me *ever*. He said I didn't say I was going to eat when I did. He never chooses to hear me. Sometimes I want to scream, *Listen to me!* while doing an Irish jig in front of his face and see if he looks up. Sometimes I feel completely invisible. I got over it and ate my lunch. It may have been because I wasn't feeling well, but everyone was pissing me off. |
| 8:30 p.m. | **Dinner:** Cheese omelet with butter on Mom's special nutritious bread (whole grain), eight ounces of water, and some Dr. Brown's cream soda.

Amount: I ate the whole sandwich. | I came home late from therapy with Dr. Blatter and between therapy, not feeling well and work, I was exhausted. After I ate, I went straight to bed. I wasn't hungry at all. |

8:45 p.m.	**Snack:** Two cups of trail mix (white chocolate chips, cashews, white chocolate pretzels, white chocolate raisins, mixed nuts, and dried fruit).	I ate it in bed while watching TV with Teddy. As I was petting him, I started to feel sorry for myself. I felt like I was failing and felt guilty. I felt bad for Teddy, too. He was stuck with me as his mom and because of that he was stuck in this fucked-up lifestyle. I know what you're thinking: he probably doesn't know the difference, he's a dog—but I swear he does! It has been very difficult for him to adjust to the house as well. He's an alpha and used to ruling his territory. He has been misbehaving and peeing everywhere to try to claim this new terrain, my parents' house, as his own. I think my mom may seriously kill him—the Napoleonic Wars are going to happen in this household with this little dog claiming his land and taking over. Remember that "the ideal Napoleonic battle was to manipulate the enemy into an unfavorable position through maneuver and deception, force him to commit his main forces and reserve to the main battle, and then undertake an enveloping attack with uncommitted or reserve troops on the flank or rear. Such a surprise attack would either produce a devastating effect on morale or force him to weaken his main battle line. Either way, the enemy's own impulsiveness began the process by which even a smaller French army could defeat the enemy's forces one by one."[11] This is a direct quote because I am not a history buff or really any kind of buff. In fact, I hate buffets and buff men—because both make me uncomfortable in different ways. But, yep, ignoring my tangent, this sounds like something Ted would do. For my mom's safety, I got to get better quickly.

Note: Although I couldn't see it at the time, this description of a Napoleonic attack may also characterize my own approach to my eating disorder.

I relapsed (abusing Colace, refer to Maudsley first relapse). The next day, I decided I had to get serious about not allowing myself to relapse again. But it was hard without a coping mechanism. Anorexia and bulimia were out of the question. Working out was not an option. I needed to find ways to feel better about this whole process. I jotted down some more questions to ask Dr. Attia. Writing helped:

Question: I think I want to know my weight to know how far I have to go, maybe. I think I need to know my weight to take some control of the situation.

---

11   Wikipedia. "Napoleonic Wars." Accessed September 6, 2016. https://en.wikipedia.org/wiki/Napoleonic_Wars

Answer: No, I was being self-destructive by wanting to know my weight. That was my eating-disordered voice asking for it. I had more control over the disease by not knowing.

Question: Can I work out again? I think it will help my stress and anxiety.

Answer: I had to wait for a certain weight and then I was allowed to work out as a reward. I couldn't use exercise as a coping mechanism just yet.

Question: Can I spend a weekend alone next weekend? Probably far-fetched because I just screwed up.

Answer: No.

Question: I am afraid of going back to my apartment for some reason... Why?

Answer: I didn't ask this question, but I knew the answer: it was because I didn't trust myself to not use laxatives on my own and go back to full-blown anorexia and bulimia.

Part of getting back on the wagon was promising to continue to journal, so I did.

DAY: Monday		
TIME	**WHAT ATE**	**HOW I FELT**
6:30 a.m.	**Breakfast:** Muesli and Fiber One mix with a splash of skim milk in a bowl. **Amount:** I ate it all.	I felt bloated and sick to my stomach. Sweat was on my sheet, blanket, neck, and arms, *everywhere*. I woke and had to change my pajama top. I felt like I was thrown into the shower with my clothes on. Going back to sleep was an arduous task. I mean, even my blanket was wet. How uncomfortable! I ate all of my cereal and felt worse. I napped on the way to work in the car, trying to catch up on sleep.

| 1:00 p.m. | **Lunch:** Cream cheese and lox on Mom's special nutritious bread (whole grain) and eight ounces of water. | I ate with the door closed, Dad across the room eating tuna fish at his desk. I sat in front of my computer, taking a ten-minute break from all the work I had to do, browsing the online gossip rags. I was extremely stressed out, anxiety creeping through my skin, replicating the feeling of what I'd imagine a bug attacking my flesh and blood to feel like. It made me quiver and the struggle to finish my sandwich was real. I needed a break.

I went to the bathroom and looked in the mirror. My face had broken out. I picked up my shirt to expose my extra-round belly. I am a greasy fat slob today. I noticed my cheeks were a little round too, so I sucked them into my teeth, trying to make them disappear. *You are so ugly.* It's never a good day when your eating-disordered voice and regular voice are basically saying the same thing. I went back to my desk and ate quickly to get it over with. |
| 9:00 p.m. | **Dinner:** Melted American cheese on a cinnamon raisin bagel and eight ounces of water. | I had a rough day. I think I am still depressed—wait, I *know* I am depressed. I am waiting for the Lexapro to work. I haven't felt good about myself in so long. I can hardly look in the mirror, not that I could before, but I feel like I am even *more* grossed out with myself. Each day is the same. It is driving me nuts. Each day is a struggle to eat, a struggle to get better. The highlight of my day is getting into bed and it being over. |

Note: I was sweating at night because my hormones were regulating as I was gaining weight. Breakouts are also from the hormone increases.

DAY: Tuesday		
TIME	WHAT ATE	HOW I FELT
6:45 a.m.	**Breakfast:** Muesli and Fiber One mix with a splash of skim milk in a bowl. **Amount:** I ate it all.	The TV I watch is hitting new lows. Oh, the Kardashians, got to love them or love to hate them. All I could think was big butts, lips, and extensions, *amazing mindless light TV*, as I ate spoonful after spoonful of my breakfast. I was still upset about everything that transpired in the past couple of days. Sometimes it is so easy to feel sad and hopeless.
1:00 p.m.	**Lunch:** Cream cheese and lox on Mom's special nutritious bread (whole grain) and eight ounces of water. **Amount:** I ate the whole sandwich.	I ate with my dad after I talked to Dr. Attia on the phone. Phone meetings are so much easier and better in general because: (a) there is no scale, meaning I don't have to get weighed, which is a *huge* plus, and (b) it's far less intimidating not seeing Dr. Attia face-to-face. Not seeing her facial expressions and hand gestures to help prove a point—her not seeing mine, or my squirming and nervous tics. I had a hard time eating at first but was able to eat after I relaxed for a little. *Deep breath in, and then exhale. Repeat.* After, I had a headache and took two Excedrins. I felt a lot better, but still so sad. I can't kick the bad feelings. I want to put my hands in the air and scream, *I surrender bad feelings.* I started singing, "Bad Feelings go away/Come again another day/" in *Rain, Rain, Go Away* nursery rhyme tune. I am losing my shit.

I didn't feel like writing the rest of the day. Every day feels so unoriginal.

Question: Everyone is a different weight; why can't I be okay health-wise at this weight? I have my period, and everything seems to be functioning properly.

Answer: It still wasn't a healthy weight. *Grrr.*

DAY: Friday		
TIME	**WHAT I ATE**	**HOW I FELT**
6:30 a.m.	**Breakfast:** Muesli and Fiber One mix with a splash of skim milk in a bowl. **Amount:** I ate it all.	I didn't sleep well because I was nervous about my appointment; even with 25 mg of trazodone added to my medicine mix to help me sleep. It's an antidepressant too. Maybe this is the little tweak I need to *finally* feel mentally better? I hope so. Tonight, I am going to take a higher dose to test it out. *You will always be miserable because you are a fucked-up person.* The day before I had weird "side effects" (quotations used because I called them side effects even though they probably weren't). Now I think it was all caused by anxiety. I was having a rough day, so I could have just felt off from that. Today I felt a lot better and didn't have any of the same "side effects"—like the headaches and unmotivated feelings that I experienced yesterday. Amazing, right?
12:00 p.m.	**Lunch:** Cream cheese and lox on Mom's special nutritious bread (whole grain) and eight ounces of water. **Amount:** I ate the whole sandwich.	I ate before my dad caught his flight to Florida. I was going to be in the office by myself for the rest of the day, so I decided to eat with him before to be safe. I didn't want to have a chance to see what I would do if I were alone and left to my own devices. "I am going to eat an early lunch with you in the room if that's okay," I said, quivering, as if a force was fighting me not to say those words. And it was; the eating disorder voice was loud, fighting me to *shut the fuck up.* Please, *of course* he is okay with it. He would actually prefer this. Especially with Mom on his back like an annoying monkey. When I am alone, I still have a strong urge to throw my lunch out. The voice screams, while figuratively pushing my fat stomach—*Dani, throw it out you fat ass.* I used to put it in a FedEx pack, seal it up, and then throw it in the garbage when no one was looking. This way the evidence was concealed, and no one would *ever* know my secret.
7:30 p.m.	**Dinner:** Cheese omelet with butter on Mom's special nutritious bread (whole grain), eight ounces of water, and some Dr. Brown's soda. **Amount:** I ate the whole sandwich.	I felt okay. I was tired because it was a long week. My dad went to Florida for the weekend because he had a business wedding. My mom was supposed to go with him but didn't because she *had* to stay with me. I felt bad and still feel bad about that. *You are ruining their lives.* I came home a pasty pale white from the car ride. I get awful motion sickness—being in the back seat of a car is absolute torture for me. I started sweating and felt a little dizzy. I lay down in the backseat, praying I wouldn't throw up. Then the nausea hit hard and fast, and I prayed a little harder. I hate that feeling. *But you would lose calories.* When I got home, I closed my eyes in my mom's bed for a little with her as we watched, more like listened, to an episode of *The Housewives*. We ate soon after. I wasn't very hungry and took it slow.

| 9:45 p.m. | **Snack:** Two cups of pretzels and dried fruit.

Amount: Two full-cup loads in a cup (red plastic cup). | I had a bite of a cookie and felt like I couldn't finish it. I had a visceral reaction and I just couldn't; my palms started sweating, and my hands started shaking, leg vibrating like it hit an electric current and it was z-z-zapping through my body. I kept thinking about how it had almost no nutritional value and on top of that, was *so* fattening! I wanted to have something I felt more comfortable with, if I had to eat, thus the pretzels—I mean, there isn't nutritional value in these either, but a much lower fat content. I ate in bed while watching a movie. I was exhausted. Thank goodness it was Friday though! I needed a weekend more than anything. |

DAY: Saturday		
TIME	**WHAT ATE**	**HOW I FELT**
8:30 a.m.	**Breakfast:** Muesli and Fiber One mix with a splash of skim milk in a bowl. **Amount:** I ate it all.	I woke at 8:00 a.m. after falling asleep at 10:45 p.m. but woke multiple times in the middle of the night. I did not leave the bed, like I normally do. I was too tired to move, almost like I was stuck in my dreams. I just tossed and turned, tossed and turned, trying to find a comfortable position and then would eventually fall back into my dreams. I took a shower, washing off the sleep, and went downstairs for breakfast. I ate with my eating companion, Mom. I felt like my stomach was extra big today—size extra-large. I have become more aware of my changing body lately as I have put on more and more weight. It has been harder and harder to ignore and to feel okay with continuing eating the way I have been. I ate it anyway of course, but I didn't really want to. What choice do I really have?

| 1:00 p.m. | **Lunch:** Vegetable panini with melted cheese and eight ounces of water.

Amount: I ate three-quarters of the sandwich. | My mom and I went for manicures and pedicures. I had my first pedicure ever. Yes, you heard me right, *ever*. I was never into pampering and would feel terrible guilt if I spent time on myself. *You are superficial and don't deserve any joys*. Plus, it was kind of a waste of time. My nails would chip and then what was the point of that? I would only consider doing it more often if there was a serum to not make your nails grow. It would take time away from my studying, exercising, doing something productive. But the verdict was unanimous. It was pretty freakin' awesome. It felt *so* good, especially the massage. It was so relaxing, a little boring, but I could get used to this treatment, I thought as the nail technician applied lotion to my feet.

After that we went to the mall for lunch before seeing a movie, *The Impossible*. I felt really bad about myself before the movie and even worse after. I felt extremely bloated, fat, and overweight—any synonym of *obese* I could think of. I only had half of my sandwich and was stuffed, or at least said I was. My mom didn't think I ate enough. She cut the remaining half of the sandwich I left on my plate into another half, urging me to eat a little more. I measured it out in my mind, trying to make it not obvious, and ate the half that was smaller. It was hard. I felt uncomfortable. I felt bad. I was struggling. I really don't want to get fat!

In the beginning of this process it was easier to eat because my stomach was a bottomless pit that didn't bloat. Now I am getting curves; I am taking up more space. I am getting bigger and my whole body can't deny that—my stomach even protrudes outward. I am becoming fat... |
| 8:30 p.m. | **Dinner:** Cheese omelet with butter on Mom's special nutritious bread (whole grain), eight ounces of water, and some Dr. Brown's soda.

Amount: I ate the whole sandwich. | I felt exhausted and drained. The movie was so sad. Then my dad called with my parents' best friends. I could tell my mom wanted to be there. I felt horrible. I was the reason she wasn't with them. *You are a burden*.

They took a picture with a little sign that said *we miss you* and sent it to my mom. They were sweet, and I felt bad she was stuck with me. I feel bad that *they* are stuck with me as their daughter. *You are a disappointment*.

I ate because I wanted to get into bed. I wasn't hungry at all and still felt fat and guilty for my stupid feelings, especially after seeing *real* problems like in the movie we just saw. I want to disappear. I should have thought a little harder before making my decision to get better that night. |

| 10:00 p.m. | **Snack:** One cup of trail mix (white chocolate chips, cashews, white chocolate pretzels, white chocolate raisins, mixed nuts, and dried fruit). | I ate it in bed to make my mom happy. I felt bad because she gave me a great day, and I felt insecure about myself during the entirety of it. She didn't really notice, only suspected it a little bit at some points. It was hard for me to eat lunch, and when I came home from the movie, she told me to swear on her life that I was good, and I could never swear on her and lie. She knows that. I was trying to avoid answering. I finally told her that I was having a hard day, but I was fine. She let it go, and I was relieved. I didn't want to talk about it anymore. I hated talking about my feelings almost more than being force-fed. |

DAY: Sunday

TIME	WHAT I ATE	HOW I FELT
9:00 a.m.	**Breakfast:** Muesli and Fiber One mix with a splash of skim milk in a bowl. **Amount:** I ate it all.	I woke feeling rested. My mom worked out while I stayed in bed. I wanted to work out too, *so badly,* but I am not allowed to yet. It is frustrating, and I am so jealous of her. I could hear the echoes of the TV and the elliptical machine from the basement through the vents. I pined for the sweat and the endorphin rush. I started doing crunches in bed, to feed the urge. I know I am not supposed to, but I did. My body is feeling better since after the seizure. I can physically work out again. I just am waiting on the okay from Dr. Attia. Hint, hint, if you are reading this and want to make my week... When we had breakfast, there was only enough milk left for a little more than one bowl full. I poured it into my bowl and poured the little bit left into the sink. My mom accused me of pouring my cereal out into the sink when I didn't. I am really trying, but she's going crazy with her paranoia. She's like the mean cop on a power trip that everyone wants to avoid on the street, except she has good intentions. Oh, and I can't seem to avoid her. She realized I didn't lie and apologized when she checked the disposal. Yes, she had to check the disposal over my word! I was a bit annoyed. I understood where she was coming from, but I have been trying so hard to gain back her trust ever since my laxative slip. I let it go and ate what I'd poured.

| 1:00 p.m. | **Lunch:** A chunky chicken salad sandwich on whole-wheat bread.

Amount: I ate three-quarters of it. | I ate half of the sandwich, and my mom forced me to eat more. I felt overstuffed and bloated—I didn't want the other half, but she forced me to eat some, and then I felt even worse. It was a big sandwich filled with a lot of chicken salad, raisins, and lettuce. I felt so uncomfortable after. I wanted to cry. I could literally feel the fat cells in my skin crawling to fill the open crevices of my body. Claiming their territory.

When I got home, I went into the bathroom in my parents' room. They have a mirror the size of the entire bathroom wall. No exaggeration. I looked at my reflection and examined myself. I saw a huge bloated stomach and a big cottage-cheese-infused-butt looking back at me. I felt so horrible and gross. I felt like I wanted my old life back and my old body back. I pulled up my sweatpants and left the bathroom as quick as I could, but not quick enough to erase that horrible image etched in my mind. |
| 8:30 p.m. | **Dinner:** Cheese omelet with butter on Mom's special nutritious bread (whole grain), eight ounces of water, and some Dr. Brown's soda.

Amount: I ate the whole sandwich.

Snack: Two cups of pretzels and dried fruit. | I had a breakdown shortly after looking in that funhouse-like mirror and couldn't stop the tears. I felt so out of control, anxious, and like I couldn't do this anymore. I wanted everything to go back to how it was, even if that meant being sick with anorexia. I couldn't stand that fat person looking back at me in the mirror. I don't know why I care about my body shape. I don't know why it upsets me. I was never the girl who cared about clothes, makeup, or anything superficial. I don't even relate to people who are focused on things like that—they bother me. *I bother me. I hate the person I have become.*

I cried so much that my mom had to call Dr. Attia to convince me I was going to be okay. She said my stomach protruding abnormally was from malnutrition, like those little kids from third-world countries in the commercials about poverty with the sad eyes and big round bellies. It would go back to normal as my weight was restored. That remark made me feel a little better, not much though. This whole situation is so messed up. I would just have to avoid mirrors for a while. That is, if she wasn't lying. |

Note: My stomach grew out and round at first because of malnutrition. This is normal during the refeeding process in someone who is extremely underweight.

DAY: Tuesday		
TIME	WHAT ATE	HOW I FELT
6:40 a.m.	**Breakfast:** Muesli and Fiber One mix with a splash of skim milk in a bowl.	I ate, but I was still questioning this entire process. I felt really lost. I wanted to be done with all of this already. I felt like a mouse that got stuck trying to get cheese in a mousetrap—hemmed in. I would have rather eaten the mouse poison; at least then I wouldn't feel *so* stuck.
1:00 p.m.	**Lunch:** Peanut butter and jelly on Mom's special nutritious bread (whole grain) and eight ounces of water. **Amount:** I ate the whole sandwich.	I ate with the door closed. My dad was waiting for me to eat so we could eat together at 12 p.m.; that's when he was hungry. At 12:20 p.m., I could tell what he was doing, which was trying to be nice, but I got annoyed because I felt so much pressure. I insisted, in an annoyed tone, that he please do his own thing. He ate while doing work, which is what he used to do. I hate that he always draws attention to my problem. I feel like some kind of pet that has to eat or do anything when someone tells me to—on command. I am tired of it. A while later, I ate even though I wasn't hungry. After I ate, I apologized to my dad for getting annoyed. He was waiting for me, and it was really a sweet gesture. I explained it was because I was feeling extra anxious and insecure today that I freaked out. He replied, "But you look good," and made a hand gesture that meant my face looked full by pointing at his cheeks. *Seriously?* "Thanks, good move, Dad," I said, angry all over again. I told him a million times that those comments upset me, and he can't seem to help himself and feels compelled to say them. It's like he prefers me upset and thinks it's laughable to exacerbate my anxiety. It is just too hard to handle sometimes. I don't understand him. I want to be done or on the last step of this process. I don't get where this is going. I am still a mess. I am just a bigger mess. What does everyone want me to be? A gigantic mess? I had a lot of work to do so I went back to it.

9:20 p.m.	**Dinner:** Steamed shrimp with mixed vegetables and brown rice. **Amount:** I ate it all.	I was really hungry. When I was eating the first piece of shrimp, I didn't chew it well and started choking. As it slid to the back of my throat, I couldn't breathe and motioned to my throat with my hands—the universal sign for "Fuck, I am choking...help me."
		My dad jumped up from his chair and put his arms around me, giving me the Heimlich. The shrimp jumped out of my throat and into the air. I saw the small red and white shrimp bounce like a fish out of water across the table. After all I had been through, could you imagine if I died choking on a shrimp? What a complete waste.
		My mom freaked out and yelled at me not to take such big bites. She couldn't do anything but break down into tears. She had had enough.
		"You are going to be the death of me," she said. After all she had been through, all she could do was stand up in place, stunned. She sat back down in her seat.
		"Now please cut your shrimp into smaller pieces." Tears were still flowing down her face. She was out of breath and tied her hair up into a tight ponytail.
		She has been on the edge of her seat with anxiety about me lately. I don't blame her. I couldn't imagine being in her shoes.
		I got up from my seat, giving her a hug, trying to comfort her, patting her on the back. "I am okay, Mom, I promise. I'm sorry."
		She looked at me again. "Death of me," she repeated, rubbing her teary eyes.
		At least I learned a lesson from this. I have to remember to cut my shrimp into smaller pieces. Duly noted.

I had a meeting with Dr. Attia and my parents that Wednesday night. Here was my takeaway—*Whoa.* They talked about me as if I wasn't sitting next to them like the dumbfounded idiot I felt like. The questions were directed around me: "How is Danielle doing?" to my parents. "Dani seems to be doing well," back to Dr. Attia. "Danielle is right here!" I wanted to scream. *She can speak English and understands it pretty proficiently too!*

This was the first appointment for all three of us. It was a little over a month into recovery, so it was time to meet as a team. Like Ren and Stimpy used to sing and bump butts to "Happy Happy Joy Joy"— *not!* I felt like I was watching my very own parent-teacher conference. And boy, I'd have done anything to be anywhere else in the world! Even eat an ice cream sundae. Seriously.

I needed to defend myself. I didn't get to share my side. Here is what I wrote:

My dad said at the meeting that I know him better than he knows himself. Fact, I can agree with that. He made that point to say he knows me better than I know myself. Wrong, that is false; no one really knows me; I don't even totally know me. He doesn't know how to handle my personality at all. If he knew me, he would know that breaking me down in a fight isn't a way to get through to me. That yesterday, when he instigated our fight, saying I looked healthier and gesturing at my face, knowing he was going to upset me, his goal was to try to get my "anxiety and anger" out. If it came out, it would go away, and I wouldn't think about it anymore, in his mind. Another fact, I don't work like that! That's how he works!

He knows that I spiraled initially when someone commented on the fact that I gained weight in my face, but it looked good. So, no, he does not know me that well if he thinks a comment like that would help me in any way. I hold onto every word as my self-hate seeps in even more.

My mom was fine in the session. I am just frustrated because it felt like a pump-up motivation session for my parents. I don't understand why my presence was even necessary. I felt like a child, but maybe that is the reason Maudsley is more common with adolescents.

The good takeaways: I was doing well with my weight gain and thus I was catapulted into Phase II of Maudsley. I would now be allowed to take more control over my eating, which was exciting. I would be able to make more food choices; however, my parents would still have to monitor my portions and intake. Basically, they still had power of veto. I guess it was our own system of checks and balances. They could shut down the eating disorder voice if they saw it was getting too powerful.

Also, Dr. Attia finally gave me the "okay" to start yoga. We are slowly making forward movements in this process. I think these are well-deserved rewards.

Note: I was allowed to start yoga because I had gained enough weight to be rewarded with exercise at this point. It was a slow start. I wasn't allowed to do any other form of exercise because my doctor wanted to see how my body reacted to the yoga first; then I would be allowed to add the elliptical machine, and so on.

This was the same with choosing foods. I was allowed to choose my cuisines now, but if my weight started to drop, that privilege would be taken away and given back to my parents.

DAY: Friday		
TIME	**WHAT I ATE**	**HOW I FELT**
6:30 a.m.	**Breakfast:** Muesli and Fiber One mix with a splash of skim milk in a bowl. **Amount:** I ate it all.	I was so exhausted. This had been a rough week, but I think I say that *every* week. I took a shower and then ate breakfast with my mom. She got mad at me because I still have to feel how deep the cereal is to make myself comfortable eating it. "That's not normal," was her response. "Clearly, I am not normal when it comes to food, if that wasn't established yet. Another point, if I could pour my own cereal, I would know how much was in it and this wouldn't be a problem to begin with," I cheekily said. My parents unfortunately still determine the amount I eat. "Well, if you are still feeling how much cereal is in the bowl, that means you are not ready to make those kinds of decisions." I repeated that if I poured my own, it wouldn't be an issue. She didn't answer. We were going in circles. It wasn't worth a fight—over cereal! We didn't talk about it further.
1:00 p.m.	**Lunch:** Cream cheese and jelly on Mom's special nutritious bread (whole grain) and eight ounces of water. **Amount:** I ate the whole sandwich.	I ate with the door closed while reading a gossip blog on the internet. I had a lot of work and things on my mind, but I took the ten-minute break, calmed down, and then ate.

| 8:30 p.m. | **Dinner:** Grilled fillet of salmon with spinach and mashed potatoes.

Amount: I ate half of a big fillet, all of the sautéed spinach, and a couple bites of the mashed potatoes. | I went out for dinner with my parents. My parents are very social beings and like to eat out a lot so my life with them consists of a lot of dinners out. I decided I wanted to try something different. I made it a point to do that because I have to start breaking away from the monotony of my meals to really get better. My mom lets me select my foods now, but if she doesn't approve, I can't have it. Before she was selecting meals for me, but I had negotiating power. With the progression into Phase II of Maudsley, I have more influence.

It was really enjoyable. It was hard to eat at first, but once I started, I was fine. The only real hurdle was eating the mashed potatoes and, trust me, when eating mashed potatoes "the struggle is real" *always*. My mom tried them, taking that thick yellowy substance from my plate with a fork and putting it into her mouth, saying, "These are good," and then eyed me like "monkey see, monkey do," taste it too.

As the children's song goes, "the monkey does the same as you," so—I had a small bite. I liked the taste, but I only had two or three more bites because I felt really uncomfortable eating it, knowing all the fat and butter that was on them. My parents told me I did well. *Good pet monkey.* |
| 10:45 p.m. | **Snack:** One cup of pretzels and dried fruit.

Amount: One full-cup load in a cup (red plastic cup). | I ate it in bed before I went to sleep. I don't try dessert at restaurants because I really don't feel comfortable eating fattening desserts like ice cream, cake, etc. There is something about the empty calories and fat that irks me. Plus, they were always labeled as "bad" foods. It is also easier for me to eat at home. When I am eating something like dessert, I would rather be in a place where I have no anxiety, like my bed. |

DAY: Saturday		
TIME	**WHAT I ATE**	**HOW I FELT**
8:30 a.m.	**Breakfast:** Muesli and Fiber One mix with a splash of skim milk in a bowl. **Amount:** I ate it all.	I ate while talking to my mom. I was hungry and gobbled it up. I have been having thoughts about how messed up my mind was before the seizure. My thoughts about my family and everything were so warped, and I really have come to realize how much I need to change. I don't want to go back to that dark place. I believed my mom and dad didn't care about me—how delusional is that? The ones who are doing everything for me right now. I want a new life. I *really* want this.

1:20 p.m.	**Lunch:** Huge mixed vegetable, portabella, and melted cheese wrap. **Amount:** I ate the whole wrap.	I was so hungry today, ravenous, I felt like Garfield inhaling lasagna. I am due to get my period in two days so that may have been the reason. I ate the whole big wrap at the restaurant. My mom tried to get me to eat the French fries at one point, but I couldn't. *Those deep-fried cut potatoes will turn your ass into cellulite. Your butt is already disgusting,* was all I could hear. I was still hungry though. I was slow with the first half of the wrap—taking my time because I enjoyed it and didn't want it to be done. Also thinking if I ate slower, I would not eat as much. Wrong! My hunger drove me to say *fuck it,* and I started to eat the second half of the wrap. I did it without alcohol or anything to ease my anxiety—I was just really hungry, so I kept on eating—*nom, nom, nom.* By the time I was done, I felt full but not overstuffed. We went home, and I made sure to put on my sweats in my room and not in the bathroom because I did not want to see my stomach in the big wall-to-wall mirror and make myself upset when I was feeling so good today.

8:40 p.m.	**Dinner:** Cream cheese and lox on Mom's special nutritious bread (whole grain) and eight ounces of water. **Amount:** I ate the whole sandwich.	My mom and dad went out for dinner, and I was left home alone. My mom wouldn't let me make anything on my own, so she made a sandwich before she went out and left it out on the table in a plastic bag for me to eat when I was ready. This was the first time they let me eat without having a watchful eye over me. I told her I would be fine, but still had some anxiety over it. Of course, I didn't express this to her. I used to rip up bread and flush it down the toilet to make it look like I ate something, when I didn't:

"Dan, what did you end up eating for dinner last night?" my mom asked, peering at the food in the refrigerator. "I had a peanut butter and jelly sandwich," I would lie. I would really take two slices of bread and flush them down the toilet in little pieces. This way, if she looked at the bread in the fridge, she would see pieces of the loaf were missing and think I was telling the truth. If she doubted me and looked in the garbage, no bread there. I thought I was so clever.

I had to start trusting myself if I wanted to go back to my apartment and be truly healthy on my own. I told her to make cream cheese and lox because I knew I was comfortable with it and could eat it even when I was not very hungry.

I took my medications at 7:30 p.m. to help with my unease, plus I wanted to go to bed at a normal time. I decided to watch a TV show while I was eating my sandwich to distract me and took my time. I had thoughts about throwing it out or flushing it down the toilet, and I easily could have, but I kept on eating it instead. Before I knew it, it was done. I was making progress. I was eating on my own, despite the voice urging me to *put down the fucking sandwich, you fucking fat ass. Flush it. Flush it.* No.

DAY: Sunday		
TIME	**WHAT I ATE**	**HOW I FELT**
8:30 a.m.	**Breakfast:** Muesli and Fiber One mix with a splash of skim milk in a bowl. **Amount:** I ate nothing.	I could not eat anything. I felt sick and nauseated. I think it was because I was getting my period. My mom was annoyed at my lack of appetite. She was actually pissed. "You know, Dan, I am really annoyed at you. You could at least have a couple of bites," she said, her hands on her hips, eyes stern. I just couldn't do it today. I don't know why she took it so personally.
1:20 p.m.	**Lunch:** Turkey, mozzarella, lettuce, and tomato wrap. **Amount:** I ate half of the wrap.	I ate while watching TV. I wasn't hungry and still did not feel well. My stomach was really bothering me. I sat with the heating pad on high blast.
8:00 p.m.	**Dinner:** Turkey, mozzarella, lettuce, and tomato wrap. **Amount:** I ate half of the wrap.	I ate the other half of the wrap because it was so big I couldn't finish it at lunch. I was really tired after and went into bed early.
9:00 p.m.	**Snack:** Two cups of pretzels, dried fruit, and graham crackers. **Amount:** Two full-cup loads in a cup (red plastic cup).	I ate them in bed while watching TV before I fell asleep. I was so worn out. This process has been so exhausting. The fact that all I am focusing on is food is exhausting. The fact that I am being monitored is exhausting. Treatment has been just as consuming as the disease itself. At least it feels that way. Every which way I turn, food is there. In the looks and expressions of my parents' faces, to the cereal I pour myself now, to the menus and stress over sauces that add up to calories at restaurants—it's all about food. That's exhausting.

DAY: Monday		
TIME	**WHAT I ATE**	**HOW I FELT**
6:30 a.m.	**Breakfast:** Muesli and Fiber One mix with a splash of skim milk in a bowl. **Amount:** I ate the whole bowl.	I was hungry. I ate the bowl and felt full. I had a good weekend. I was feeling relatively fine, compared to how I used to be. I think that's a healthy comparison to make, and it makes me feel a little better.
1:00 p.m.	**Lunch:** Vegetarian wrap with roasted vegetables, fresh mozzarella, and balsamic vinegar in an herb wrap. **Amount:** I ate half of the wrap.	I am starting to feel a little more at ease with variety. I am trying really hard at least. I ordered off the menu from takeout at work instead of opting for the sandwiches my mom makes for me. I was given a menu and looked at it, thinking, *What would be healthy and nutritious?* I chose a veggie wrap because veggies are healthy and not high in calories. I let the mozzarella cheese be in it for the fat, since I need to still gain weight. I know, I shouldn't think about calories, but I do when making these decisions. Anyway, it was really good. I had a hard time once my dad started making suggestions about what I should eat the next day and the day after and what I could do, should do, etc. I wanted to scream "LEAVE ME ALONE!" Can't we get through this day and this meal first? He continued to go on *and on* about how I can't eat what I was having every day because it was repetitive. We discussed this with Dr. Attia at our meeting on Wednesday. Oh, and apparently since then Dad has become an eating disorder specialist. At first the monotony in my food choices were okay because we were focused solely on gaining weight, but now I needed to start varying more because we were focusing on a healthy lifestyle change I could adapt to after I hit my target weight. There needs to be variety in diet in order to be healthy and not have disordered eating. I was annoyed my dad was pushing me. Okay, I do eat veggie wraps a lot, I get it, but I never got one at work! He doesn't understand baby steps. He would love to just shake and fix me. I'd love it if he could too! *Trust me, I am all about the easy fix.* I nodded in agreement, but I nodded mostly to shut him up. I think he was trying to make a point, but he chose the wrong time because I was actually trying something new by ordering in at work myself. I didn't want to continue talking about it while I ate. It made it harder for me to eat when I thought too much about my feelings. I am really trying to push myself out of my comfort zone to the best of my ability.

8:30 p.m.	**Dinner:** A slice of vegetable pizza and a bowl of warm shrimp pasta. **Amount:** I ate a lot of the warm shrimp pasta and the whole slice of pizza. **Snack:** two cup loads of cashews.	I felt really good after yoga. I am surprised I liked it. My mom and I did it together. Our instructor isn't bad to look at either which is a nice workout bonus. *Hey there, Mr. Handsome! Purr.* Kidding! Kind of. He was very sweet and taught us basic yoga poses. I liked warrior pose, because I do feel like a warrior every day lately. Waking up to battle food and conquer it multiple times a day.

I was really hungry after our exercise session. I ate with my mom and dad at the kitchen table. I didn't even order the warm shrimp pasta but had some anyway. I wanted to try it because it looked good. I hesitated at first, but then once I had some, I put some more in a bowl that I finished.

On another note, today my dad yelled at me because he was stressed out. Instead of getting mad at myself or taking it personally, I just kind of explained to him why his behavior was wrong, how ridiculous what he was yelling about was, and laughed it off because it didn't make sense. How mature, *right?* A little bit later, he apologized because he realized he was wrong. I knew he was just stressed and that usually made me feel tense, but it didn't this time. I told him it was okay, and it was *really* okay for the first time ever! I didn't feel bad about it or take it to heart. I rationalized it and helped him out with other tasks at work. We worked together and accomplished more that way. How very *Full House* perfect of us, *right?* Danny Tanner and DJ have nothing on my dad and me.

I find that it is easier for me to eat and try new things when I am able to handle conflict. I usually take things personally and am not able to eat because I am so upset at myself. Today I expressed my feelings instead of holding them in, and, by letting them out, the conflict was fixed and I didn't feel the need to punish myself. It was a better resolve.

DAY: Tuesday		
TIME	WHAT I ATE	HOW I FELT
7:00 a.m.	**Breakfast:** Muesli and Fiber One mix with a splash of skim milk in a bowl. **Amount:** I ate the whole bowl.	I slept really well. I was feeling sore from yoga yesterday, but the best I have felt in a really long time—longer than I can remember. I like feeling sore, it makes me feel like I am actually using my body. Wait, correction, actually using my body for something besides eating! Hallelujah! I ate the bowl of cereal with that thought.
1:00 p.m.	**Lunch:** Honey mustard chicken wrap with Roma tomatoes and mesclun greens in an herb and garlic wrap.	I ate with my dad. I was starving. I am just trying to let my hunger drive me lately. I wanted to change up my routine again and went for what I was in the mood for, which was the honey mustard chicken wrap. It was really good, and I ate the whole wrap. This week is the best I have felt in a long time. That's a bold statement, but I feel like maybe I have a chance. I feel like maybe all of the antidepressants have kicked in because I feel calmer toward everything or maybe it's me (which I hope, but either/or, I just want the feeling to stay and keep on improving).
9:30 p.m.	**Dinner:** Cheese omelet with butter on plain buttered bagel. **Amount:** I ate the whole sandwich.	My parents went out for dinner, and I got dropped off at home after therapy later in the night. I was hungry, but exhausted. I was also a little upset by some topics Dr. Blatter brought up. I hate verbalizing when things are bothering me and right now *everything* is bothering me. I prefer shutting completely down, *especially* when things are terrible. I would prefer a vow of silence—the Buddhist monk way. Unfortunately, I don't think that's an option.

I relapsed with the natural laxatives (refer to second relapse Maudsley chapter).

DAY: Wednesday

TIME	WHAT I ATE	HOW I FELT
6:30 a.m.	Breakfast: Muesli and Fiber One mix with a splash of skim milk in a bowl. **Amount:** I ate the whole bowl.	I didn't feel well from the laxatives I took yesterday. My mom had found them because my stomach was bad and sadly her instant thought and instinct became that I must be making myself sick again. She was right, *unfortunately.* I got them on my way to Dr. Blatter once again. This time my stash didn't last as long though. I had them for less than twenty-four hours when my mom found them. She should be a detective, I swear! I guess it's pretty easy to detect me though. Simple statistics, Dani has a bad stomachache, there is an extremely high probability that she is taking laxatives again. *Bingo!*
1:45 p.m.	**Lunch:** Vegetarian wrap with roasted vegetables, fresh mozzarella, and balsamic vinegar in an herb wrap. **Amount:** I ate half of the wrap.	I still didn't feel well. I ate half the wrap and was finished. I was also nervous for my session with Dr. Attia tonight, which made it harder to eat. I knew I screwed up once again, and I didn't know how she was going to take it. Once, she was compassionate, but two times? I hated that I had to tell her too. I wished she could just read it in here. It was a terrible punishment for my petty crime. My parents said I would have to tell her about my slip myself, and they were going to *make sure* I did. I would have preferred jail time.
8:30 p.m.	**Dinner:** Cheese omelet with butter on plain buttered bagel **Amount:** I ate the whole sandwich.	I ate it all. I screwed up badly and wanted to try to never be tempted to take laxatives ever again. Hearing Dr. Attia call it a *relapse* made me cringe because of how well I thought I was doing. But it was that—a cringe, hand-covering-face-emoji relapse. She was very nice and understanding about it though. I think she was the only one who didn't feel betrayed by my actions. I just wanted to take back some control. I know I did it in the wrong way, but this has always been my coping mechanism. I don't want to keep making myself sick forever. I want to be a good example for my future, if-I-have-a-future, kids. I am also tired of being monitored and infantilized. I feel like a child. I need to get my act together if I want to be treated like the adult I am.
9:30 p.m.	**Snack:** One cup of honey wheat pretzels with mixed dried fruit.	I ate them in bed before I went to sleep, thinking hard about my newfound laxative sobriety.

I jotted down a list of healthy coping mechanisms I could replace laxatives with that night when I couldn't sleep and was sick of counting sheep—baa one, baa two... Damn this, it doesn't work:

A List of Healthy Activities That Make Me Feel Good/Why:

Exercise: Running on the treadmill, my feet slam up and down. My hair bounces against my neck. I can hear the machine roar, a symphony of squeaks, whines, and screeches. Once I am in the groove, my running groove, none of that bothers me. Sweat pours down my neck, into my sports bra, and against my stomach. I listen to music, and all I do is run, like nothing can stop me. P!nk blaring in my ears, inspiring me. I can feel my heart beating loudly to the music vibrating through my ears. It's not about calories; it's about feeling refreshed and alive, at peace.

Elliptical or Spinning: Same feeling as the treadmill.

Writing: Getting my thoughts on paper feels so good, a positive way of coping. Writing about what has happened has been a powerful way to come to terms with everything and accept the outcome that, yes, I was anorexic/bulimic, and I am in recovery right now, and that's okay. Writing has been cathartic and makes it easier to discuss my issues day-to-day and accept my truth, preventing me from falling back. I wake up dying to let out my feelings, and not in a self-destructive way. I get my grubby thoughts out on paper, cleansing my mind and soul. No one is judging what I say or do. It can be my own private sanctuary and that's what I love about it.

Blogging: All the benefits of writing minus no one is judging you, 'cause everyone is! But, honestly, who the fuck cares? My new 'tude toward things like this is that maybe you can start a positive movement and help someone. You can get immediate feedback. Besides, criticism and Wheaties are the breakfast of champions, they say. Blogging (I was still debating about starting one at this point) will give me a much thicker skin and a new perspective—maybe even some purpose.

Talk to My Support System: A support system is a network of people who provide an individual with practical or emotional support. I find that talking to my support team about things is a healthy way to clear my mind and gives me a fresh, unbiased perspective. I think it is very important for people in recovery to have a group of people, or at least a person, they can count on for advice and help when they are struggling.

DAY: Thursday		
TIME	**WHAT I ATE**	**HOW I FELT**
6:30 a.m.	**Breakfast:** Muesli and Fiber One mix with a splash of skim milk in a bowl. **Amount:** I ate the whole bowl.	I slept horribly. I was up from 1:30 to 3:00 a.m. watching TV and thinking. I was thinking about my life and how I am disappointed with where I am. People I went to high school with are getting engaged, married, having babies, or at least have boyfriends/partners. If not that, at least they are fucking living on their own. I ate my cereal and decided from here on out, I am going to pour my own cereal. This is how I am going to slowly take back control—one cereal bowl at a time. I am going to stop hurting myself and regain my independence. This is what Dr. Attia is banking on, and this is what I will do. At least this is the moment's plan.
1:00 p.m.	**Lunch:** Vegetarian wrap with roasted vegetables, fresh mozzarella, and balsamic vinegar in an herb wrap. **Amount:** I ate half of the wrap.	I ate with the door open. I didn't care if anyone made comments about my eating. No one did. I hope this has become the new normal. I wasn't invited to my dad's two meetings, which upset me, but I didn't tell him that. I have always tried to prove to him that I am meeting-worthy. I have voiced this, and he always made up an excuse (using my lack of getting dressed up properly for work: makeup, hair, and clothes) or said I simply don't belong there. I had come in to work in the past with my hair and makeup done, wearing business-casual nice clothes, and I still wasn't allowed. I convinced myself I didn't belong because he was ashamed of me: I wasn't pretty enough, smart enough, etc. I think my thoughts were my anorexia speaking to me. Telling me that no one thought I was enough, *not even* my dad. These would be triggers for me to starve myself or binge and purge. Truth is, as I have gotten better, I have realized that I really just don't belong at some of these meetings, but I still can't stop hearing the voices telling me it's because I am a disappointment. Why do I have to take everything out on myself?
8:00 p.m.	**Dinner:** Salmon fillet in a tomato sauce with vegetables. **Amount:** I ate half the fillet and all the vegetables.	We went out for dinner for my mom's birthday. I was a little upset about some things today, but I let them go. I didn't want to ruin her birthday like I have ruined everything else. I wanted it to be special for her like she tried to make my birthday. I ordered the fillet of salmon. It came with a lot of sauce on it. At first, I was a little afraid of that drenched fish, but then once I dug into it, I was fine, and it was good. It was a really nice family dinner. My dad and I had a talk before bed about my progress at work and treatment. It was positive, but I couldn't sleep and was a little hungry. I had a cup of cereal before bed like a normal person who was snacking; crazy, *right*?

DAY: Friday		
TIME	**WHAT I ATE**	**HOW I FELT**
6:30 a.m.	**Breakfast:** Kellogg's Fruit and Yogurt, Raisin Bran, and Fiber One mix with a splash of skim milk in a bowl. **Amount:** I ate the whole bowl.	My mom was on the way out because she was going to a friend's surgery. I came down to the kitchen and gave her a kiss on the cheek and said "*Au revoir*" in my best French accent. She smiled at me. "Have a good day, freakazoid," she said as she slammed the door behind her. "Oui, oui," I answered back. These were the only "two" words I knew in French. Anyway, there I was, alone for breakfast for the first time in a long time. I went into the cabinet looking for cereal. I saw Raisin Bran, Kellogg's Fruit and Yogurt, and Fiber One. I grabbed them all out and poured them one by one into the same bowl. I was making a mix, a cocktail of sorts. I poured a nice amount of milk in (I was still pretending to be French since I was in chef mode and some of the best chefs are French, so my instinct was to transform into Raymond Blanc in that moment, *naturally*) and shook it, mixing it all together. I even poured extra because I was hungry. I sat down at the kitchen table and ate spoonful after spoonful, no problem. It was surprisingly easy to eat. I can now eat on my own like a pro. I proved it to myself in that moment, which was most important of all. I gave myself two Michelin stars and two thumbs up on my all-around performance.
1:00 p.m.	**Lunch:** Vegetarian wrap with roasted vegetables, fresh mozzarella, and balsamic vinegar in an herb wrap. **Amount:** I ate half of the wrap	Today was the first of the month, February first. I have been in treatment for about two months now. It was extra busy in the office. I was really in the mood for this veggie wrap. I ate with the door open and then went back to work. I had a lot on my mind. I was excited for the weekend and to get home tonight because I had yoga again. I was thrilled to get some body movement in, even if it's not my favorite form of exercise. It feels good to move and break a sweat. As they say, "Beggars can't be choosers," so I am just happy to be getting the chance to work out.

| 8:00 p.m. | **Dinner:** Broiled tilapia with sautéed spinach and corn. **Amount:** I ate most of the fish and all of the vegetables. | After yoga, my parents and I took my parents' friend out for dinner because his wife was away in Florida for the weekend. He was my date for the night. Best date I have had in a long time! Unfortunately, no sarcasm there. It was a nice time and the fish was really good. Before yoga, I was feeling a little bad about my body and myself. The workout made me feel less gross and more like a human being. Breaking a sweat and the endorphins followed by a nice shower changed my whole mood. |
| 10:30 p.m. | **Snack:** One apple and some pretzels. | I ate a healthy snack in bed before I fell asleep. I opted for something healthy and low-calorie because I felt better with the thought of those items sitting in my belly all night long. *You are worthless.* No, I am not... |

DAY: Saturday

TIME	WHAT ATE	HOW I FELT
8:30 a.m.	**Breakfast:** Kellogg's Fruit and Yogurt, Cap'n Crunch, and Fiber One mix with a splash of skim milk in a bowl. **Amount:** I ate the whole bowl.	I was feeling hungry this morning after doing a little bit of morning yoga. I took it upon myself to go downstairs to the basement and practice different yoga poses on my own. Exercising is really helping me feel a lot better. I can't wait to really exert myself besides doing yoga. I want to stick with it for now though because it is the only thing I am allowed to do. I poured the cereal myself again. I am not thinking about calories. I am starting to think about what is healthy and good for my body. I want to be a healthy person. I am eating when I am hungry and eating until I feel satisfied now.
2:00 p.m.	**Lunch:** Vegetarian wrap with roasted vegetable, fresh mozzarella, and balsamic vinegar in a wrap.	We went to the diner on Route 4 that has the best wraps. I had the veggie wrap, but it was so big that I only ate half and was completely stuffed. I felt good after.

8:00 p.m.	**Dinner:** Surf and turf and sautéed spinach. **Amount:** I ate half of the huge fillet and about half of the lobster.	We went out for dinner with my mom's cousin and her husband at the Palm. They are such nice people, and it's always good seeing them. It is easy to go out and eat even in public with people like them. I have become the official plan crasher/third wheel, but I don't think they cared. We stayed until 11:00 p.m., shutting the restaurant down, just talking. It was a really good time.

Sunday: I skipped the day of writing, but I did binge on trail mix Sunday night.

DAY: Monday		
TIME	**WHAT ATE**	**HOW I FELT**
7:00 a.m.	**Breakfast:** Kellogg's Fruit and Yogurt, and Fiber One mix with skim milk in a bowl. **Amount:** I ate the whole bowl.	I poured it. I felt a little gross from last night's binge; I had four cup-loads of trail mix! I did yoga poses and played a little bit of soccer, kicking a ball around and running after it, to feel better, before my dad started getting ready for work. No, I am not approved for soccer or running, but I couldn't care less; plus, it worked. I was hungry by the time I had breakfast, able to eat, and felt so much better. Proof I should be allowed to do any exercise I want.
1:00 p.m.	**Lunch:** Honey mustard chicken wrap. **Amount:** I ate half of the wrap	I got my period. That is what explained my hunger last night and my bloating and cramping this morning. I felt gross, but a lot better that there was a reason for it; also, a reason why I was so damn hungry last night. I ate with the door open. I don't even think about closing the door anymore unless to sometimes get a moment of sanity to myself. It is not to hide my eating habits though, so that's a big improvement.

7:30 p.m.	**Dinner:** Bronzini with grilled mixed vegetables in a white sauce. **Amount:** Half the bronzini and most of the grilled vegetables.	We went out for dinner with my parents' friends. It was a disaster for me. First, my mom didn't approve of my order. I first wanted "the sole plain" and was in the middle of ordering it when she interjected, "She wants the tomato sauce on it."
		"No, I don't. I am not in the mood for tomato sauce," I angrily said back to the waiter, meaning to direct that anger toward my mom.
		My dad simultaneously decided then that it was okay to make a loud suggestion. Then my parents' friends decided to suggest that I try the bronzini, so I went with that trying to get everyone to shut the fuck up!
		I wanted it all to stop. I was really embarrassed but tried to keep my composure. My mom later apologized on behalf of her and my dad, but it still hurt. My parents' friends don't know why I am home. I told my parents to tell them it was because of my eye problems, but my parents are making it pretty fucking obvious it is more than just my eyes. I guess if their friends have eyes of their own, they could tell that for themselves.
		I think during this period I would be better off at my apartment. I am doing really well and think I can do this with just my team of doctors. Living and working with my parents has become way too much. At the same time, I am a little afraid of going home for some reason. Okay, I know the reason. It is because I feel like I have nothing there and so much to build, and it frightens me. I need my independence though, and I have to start somewhere. I am twenty-six already. Nothing seems easy ever! I want to scream. So I will scream on paper AHHHHHHHH! One more time a little louder, AHHHHHHHHHHHHHHHHHHHH!! Better.

Around this time, we went on a leisure trip to Florida to visit my grandma and get out of town for a long weekend. Here's what I wrote:

Florida Trip Summary:

I was too busy with work and activities to write while I was in Miami so I thought I would jot down a quick recap. By activities, I mean hardcore relaxing while basking in the boiling beams of the sun. Yes, be completely jealous! It wasn't easy for me to relax at first because of my body hatred, which translated into all-around self-hatred like it usually does. I had black baggy Champion shorts and a white T-shirt on, making me feel uncomfortable and exposed because my body was showing more than usual. My poor white pasty virgin-to-the-sun skin turned a shade of red by the weekend's end.

Unfortunately for me, the weather in Florida is not conducive to wearing leggings and big sweaters. I was very insecure, especially since I've put on weight. On top of that, I had no idea how much weight I've put on, which killed me even more. I noticed small changes: my arms showed, but they weren't as tiny as I remembered. I had some flab that made itself a home on my upper arms. My legs had more density to them and weren't the twigs that bruised easily from drunkenly crashing into walls at night, stumbling over God knows what. Things were different in so many ways, but a good kind of different overall. I just needed to get used to it.

It's so toxic to be in hiding. It was such an all-consuming secret, and I had so much shame it would be discovered that I didn't even realize how consuming it became trying to conceal it. I don't miss that secret life at all. If I were still in hiding, I would be missing out on these past few beautiful days in paradise: Spanish-style houses and laughter with my mom.

"Mom," I said looking at her seriously on our last day, "can I stay here forever?" I added a pouty face for effect.

"Unfortunately, we all have to go back."

"Boo," I said, giving her the thumbs down.

I hadn't been to Miami in over four years, so it felt good to be back, oh, and on vacation to boot. Ted was happy to be away too. I could tell by his demeanor. He was more playful than usual, jumping up and down on me like a puppy when I got back from a boat ride or a walk on the beach. Maybe it was because I was feeling happier and he could sense it.

As far as eating went, I ate an eclectic group of foods. I had surf and turf with vegetables one night; brown rice, duck sauce, and chicken and mixed vegetables another night; and halibut with grilled mixed vegetables another night. For lunch, I had a chicken and tomato gyro with lettuce and a cucumber sauce. Another day, I had a grilled chicken sandwich on a bun with mozzarella cheese, tomato, and a pesto sauce. Another day, for lunch, I had a vegetable wrap with mixed vegetables (obviously), hummus, and mozzarella with balsamic vinegar. It was overall a nice time going away—it felt good to relax a little. The only thing that bothered me was that, even when I could relax workwise, I could never relax treatment or recovery. I need a food-cation, too! I don't think that will ever happen though. Hopefully, one day I will consider good food an essential part of a great vacation.

I only had two times where I felt really bad about myself, where I didn't want to be seen in public and wanted to hide under the covers, head under the pillow, but I got over it or got through it at least by getting up and out of bed anyway—fighting that bad feeling—pushing through the way I promised myself after reading that article in Psychology Today (that concept applies to a lot of steps in recovery). I found that doing exercise like taking a walk and then showering improved my mood. In the near future, I think I will be ready to start moving back home in small steps. I wonder what Dr. Attia will think. I would go as slow as she wants. I just need forward movements. I feel like I am okay enough. I mean, look at me, now taking long weekends to go on vacation without feeling guilty. Who would have thunk? Clearly, now I am living on the edge.

DAY: Tuesday		
TIME	**WHAT I ATE**	**HOW I FELT**
6:30 a.m.	**Breakfast:** Kellogg's Fruit and Yogurt and Fiber One mix with skim milk in a bowl.	I was feeling tired today and didn't want the day to begin. Three adults under the same roof isn't a healthy lifestyle for anyone. My mom was picking on me this morning. I can't take it anymore. At twenty-six, I am not supposed to be disciplined like a child. I don't think my parents can stand me anymore either and I don't blame them! This is not healthy. My friends (or more like peers) have lives and families of their own, and I am stuck in the worst purgatory, more like no-purge-a-tory, since purging isn't allowed, which makes this *so* much harder. I am going to now scream on paper to make myself feel better: AHHHHHHHHHH. Believe me, this paper-screaming thing helps. I swear by it.
1:00 p.m.	**Lunch:** Honey mustard chicken and lettuce in an herb wrap. **Amount:** I ate half of the wrap.	I ate it quickly and then went back to work. I had a rough day. I was feeling really down. I am ready to start the next phase where I go back to my apartment—I just need something to strive for—a date to look forward to, something concrete. I feel so lost and sad. I am unsure of everything right now and need to start rebuilding my life. I feel like everything is currently so stagnant and I am physically full because I am eating, but my life is still empty.
9:00 p.m.	**Dinner:** Six steamed vegetable dumplings, brown rice, and mixed vegetables with duck sauce. **Amount:** I ate most of it.	I waited until my mom came home from dinner because it makes her feel uncomfortable if I don't, but I told her to start getting more comfortable with the idea of me eating alone because I am doing better, and she needs to start trusting me again in order for us to proceed to the next steps: "I will wait for you to get home this time, but just warm up to the idea of me eating on my own." I paused then added, "please"—a little sugar goes a long way sometimes. I wanted her to warm up to the idea instead of just demanding it and then getting into a fight about it. I know I have put her through a lot, and it hasn't come without slips, but I finally am doing the best I have ever done in regard to food and health and feel confident enough that I know I will eat well on my own. I don't think I am afraid of being on my own anymore. Okay, I may have lied. If I am being really honest, I *do* feel afraid of being on my own. I am not afraid of the eating as much as I am afraid I will give in to the laxative temptation. Especially when I remember and reflect on the past. I don't want to go back...

There was much more to my Food & Feelings Journal—a couple of months' worth of entries—but I think you get the point. My journal entries and stories illustrate the struggles of recovering through Maudsley as an adult. Weight restoration/recovery was incredibly difficult—the most grueling, backbreaking, arduous thing I have ever overcome—emotionally as well as physically. However, if you have the right motivation and support, you can recover. Anyone can. Even me.

Resources

Every ED case is different and should be treated uniquely. My book should no way be your only source for getting well. I am not a professional on these matters, and you will need at least one as a guide on your own path to recovery. Please review the following resources to help you, a family member, or a peer get through your/ their time with anorexia, bulimia, or binge eating disorder. You cannot beat this illness alone, but recovery is more than possible with a team of support.

National Eating Disorders Association (NEDA)

NEDA is the largest not-for-profit organization in the United States working to prevent eating disorders and provide information and treatment referrals to individuals and families suffering from eating disorders.

If you are worried about a peer or family member who is suffering from an eating disorder, call the NEDA helpline, 1-800-931-2237. Live Helpline Hours: Monday through Thursday from nine to nine eastern time and Friday from nine to five eastern time.

They will guide you to helpful places to treat your eating disorder and fit your recovery to your individual needs, including any financial issues or help with interventions. They will even help you take legal action to help your loved one if necessary: http://www.nationaleatingdisorders.org/find-help-support

NEDA Navigators are volunteers who have experience navigating the complex and overwhelming systems and emotions involved with the diagnosis and process of seeking help for an eating disorder. Volunteers are trained by NEDA staff, clinical advisors, and NEDA founders to be a knowledgeable, informal source of support and guidance to those who are new to the illness:

https://www.nationaleatingdisorders.org/blog/get-the-support-you-deserve-today

The Columbia Center for Eating Disorders/Eating Disorders Clinic at the New York State Psychiatric Institute
https://www.columbiapsychiatry.org/research-clinics/eating-disorders-clinic

The Columbia Center for Eating Disorders is an internationally recognized program committed to the research and treatment of eating disorders. Founded in 1979 by Dr. B. Timothy Walsh, the Center is currently under the leadership of Dr. Evelyn Attia. Our multidisciplinary team has unparalleled expertise in cutting edge research, which is used to provide as well as develop innovative therapies.

Designated a Center of Excellence as part of a New York State initiative, our program is part of New York State Psychiatric Institute, located at Columbia University Medical Center. The unit provides comprehensive clinical services based on best practices. Our program is unique in its ability to offer treatment at no cost in exchange for participation in research.

Eating Disorders Clinic
1051 Riverside Drive
Unit 98
New York, NY 10032
646-774-8066 | edru@nyspi.columbia.edu

The Eating Disorders Clinic at the New York State Psychiatric Institute
New York State Psychiatric Institute
Eating Disorders Clinic
Unit 98
1051 Riverside Drive
NY, NY 10032
212-543-5739 | EDRU@pi.cpmc.columbia.edu

The Eating Disorder Referral and Information Center Scholarship Program
http://www.edreferral.com/scholarshipcontent.htm
Provides scholarships through funding from charitable donations.

F.R.E.E.D. (Foundation for Research and Education in Eating Disorders) Foundation
http://www.freedfoundation.org
Gail Schoenbach, NY
908-756-9260 | gailsfreedfdn@aol.com

A foundation that raises money for scholarships to help people fund treatment for eating disorders. This organization also provides support for families and patients when insurance denials block access to care.

Project Heal

https://www.theprojectheal.org/who-we-are/

Is America's strongest voice that full recovery from an eating disorder is possible and should be accessible. What began as Project HEAL's core work to fundraise and award grants for in-patient treatment, the Treatment Access Program has evolved to ensure that beneficiaries are equipped to utilize the insurance coverage they are entitled to, and that when coverage cuts out, their treatment partners ensure that you can stay in treatment as long as you need. In 2019, they partnered with The Kennedy Forum to build a model mental health parity enforcement program.

Eating Recovery Center

https://www.eatingrecoverycenter.com/about-us

Utilizes a full continuum of care, provides expert behavioral health and medical treatment for eating disorders in an environment of compassion, competence, collaboration, and integrity. It is an international center for eating disorders recovery providing comprehensive treatment for anorexia, bulimia, binge eating disorder, and other unspecified eating disorders

Nothing about eating disorders is simple, but with the right guidance, you can get well. Remember, you are beautiFULL and worth it. You deserve to live a FULL life.

Acknowledgments

Mango Publishing: None of this could have been possible without you. The day we signed a contract, I knew my book found a perfect home and your enthusiasm, support, and guidance in this process has never faltered. Thank you for believing in me and my story. Thank you for making my dream of getting a book out there to help people with eating disorders a reality. What you brought to life, is better than I could have ever imagined.

My parents: For basically *everything* (to be blunt). For letting me move in during my weight-restoration step of recovery and standing beside me through every phase of this disease and life. I wouldn't be here without your belief that I was worth fighting for. I love you both so much.

My husband: You *really* do make me believe in flying pigs. I couldn't imagine being in this good mental place without sharing it with you. I couldn't have written this book without your constant support and understanding. I know it was *very* time-consuming, so thank you, my love. Also, thank you for always knowing how to defuse me when you hear glimpses of ED and not Dani. And last but not least, for being the best father to my incredible kids. I am very lucky to have you as my partner in life.

My entire family: Thank you for supporting my recovery through the past six years and understanding my absence during my hard times. I am happy I have many more years to make up for lost time. I love you all endlessly.

My in-laws: Thank you for always supporting me. You have been a gift in my recovery and in my life.

Dr. Brett Blatter: Your help and guidance have always been above and beyond. You were a rock during my hard times and a sounding board I rely on still today.

Dr. Evelyn Attia: Thank you so much for getting me through the refeeding process. It was a difficult journey, and without you in command, we would have been lost. Also, the foreword to this book, I so appreciate you and can't thank you enough.

Teddy: My amazing dog and guardian angel. You stood by me every day as a companion, even through my loneliest and darkest days. You will forever be in my heart.

Vivienne and Diana: My beautiful daughters. You make every hard day I ever had worth it. You are my top reason why I would never go back to ED. You make me want to make the world infinitely better because you are both a part of it. I can't wait to see you both become the amazing, strong, FULL women I know you will be. Keep being you and doing whatever makes your heart sing and I will be here always to guide and support you. I love you both more than anything.

Uncle Fil: You are a gem of a human being. Thank you for your legal advice and all-around advice. I am lucky to have you in my life.

Michele Matrisciani, Betsy Robinson, and Carol Killman Rosenberg: Thank you for taking my words and asking for more. The first drafts were pitiful compared to what this book has become, and I can only thank you for asking for more from me and giving me a nice solid foundation. Also, I appreciate you talking me off the ledge at times. The industry is rough, and it was nice to have someone to vent to.

Lindsey Alexander and Emily Matchar from The Reading List: Thank you for my final edit that made my book publisher-ready and ready for the public. From the eyes of this recovering perfectionist—it wasn't easy to feel comfortable releasing this into the world—but you got me there! So thank you!

My Her View from Home Family: You have only been in my life for a short time but the amount of support I have gotten from all of you in my writing each day is overwhelming. Thank you for that. You are all women that like to inspire and encourage each other to the top. That's why I am pretty sure I found my tribe.

To everyone out there affected by eating disorders: I want you to know that recovery is possible! I promise, if you give it a real chance, soon the loud, dark, negative voices of ED will become soft, low whispers and slowly dissipate. It is so worth the fight, and you will be stronger for overcoming it. I wish all of you a FULL life.

About the Author

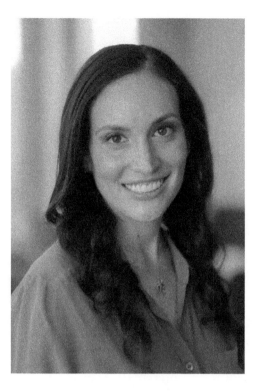

Danielle Sherman-Lazar is an eating disorder advocate, Vice President of a transportation company, and a mother to two daughters, Vivienne and Diana. She has been published on Scary Mommy, Bluntmoms, The Mighty, Eating Recovery Center, Kidspot, ellenNation, Project Heal, Love What Matters, Cafemom.com, Beating Eating Disorders, Her View From Home, Motherly, Sammiches and Psych Meds, Recovery Warriors, Kveller.com, Humorwriters.org, and That's Inappropriate. She has also contributed and has been featured on Today Parents and the *Today* show. Follow her on her blog Living a FULL Life After ED (https://livingafulllifeaftered.com/) and follow it on Facebook (https://www.facebook.com/StrivingToBeFULLeveryday/). She loves to be in touch with her readers and anyone that needs hope or guidance in eating disorder recovery. She writes about recovery from eating disorders and motherhood—a lot of time both together—her two passions in life. Danielle writes, works and lives with her family in the Tri-State area.